P9-CEE-426

Praise for Jorge Cruise and his 8-minute weight-loss plan

"Lose 2 pounds a week."
—USA Weekend

"Jorge Cruise guarantees we're going to be looking beautiful in that bathing suit."
—CNN

"See amazing results!"
—iVillage.com

"Will have you fit, firm and feeling fabulous—no sweat required."
—First for Women *magazine*

"NO trips to the gym. NO endless walking sessions. NO complicated meal plans. A science-based quickie strategy that has already helped millions of folks get slim."
—Woman's World *magazine*

"The perfect plan when you are short on time."
—Prevention *magazine*

"Jorge wants to get you super-healthy, not just super-lean."
—Fit *magazine*

"Jorge is America's newest weight-loss guru!"
—Better Nutrition *magazine*

"A must for anyone trying to lose weight and get in shape. It works!"
—Denise Austin, host of Lifetime TV's Daily Workout

"Great results in less time than it takes to shower in the morning. If you have been procrastinating about starting an exercise program, you have no more excuses."
—Kathy Smith, best-selling fitness author

"If you can't take 8 minutes out of a 24-hour day to take care of the most important person on the Earth, you are just plain lazy. Jorge will get you up and started."
—Jack LaLanne, the "Godfather of Physical Fitness" and host of the first nationally syndicated exercise show on television

"Sets you up to win!"
—Anthony Robbins, best-selling author of Unlimited Power and Awaken the Giant Within

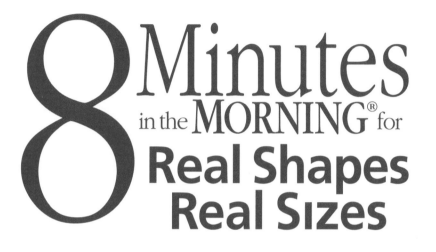

8 Minutes in the MORNING® for Real Shapes Real Sizes

8 Minutes in the MORNING® for Real Shapes Real Sizes

Specifically Designed for People Who Want to Lose 30 Pounds or More

JORGE CRUISE

The *N.Y. TIMES* BEST-SELLING AUTHOR with over 3 million online weight-loss clients

RODALE

© 2003 by Jorge Cruise, Inc.
Cover Photograph © Robert Trachtenberg
Interior Photographs © Rodale Inc.

Jorge Cruise, 8 Minutes in the Morning, The People Solution, Cruise Moves, Cruise Down Plate, and *Cruise Down* are trademarks of Jorge Cruise, Inc., and may not be used without permission.

Jorge Cruise's clothing provided by Nike, Adidas, and Hugo Boss

All rights reserved. No part of this publication may be reproduced or transmitted in any form or by any means, electronic or mechanical, including photocopying, recording, or any other information storage and retrieval system, without the written permission of the publisher.

Printed in the United States of America
Rodale Inc. makes every effort to use acid-free ∞, recycled paper ♻.

Book design by Christopher Rhoads
Food Photographer: John Hamel
Other Interior Photography: Mitch Mandel
Clothing Stylist: Christine Edmonds/REINHARD
Hair-Makeup Stylist: Colleen Kobrick
Food Stylist: Melissa DeMayo

Library of Congress Cataloging-in-Publication Data

Cruise, Jorge.
    8 minutes in the morning for real shapes, real sizes : specifically
designed for people who want to lose 30 pounds or more / Jorge Cruise.
       p.   cm.
    ISBN 1–57954–714–1   hardcover
    1. Weight loss—Popular works.   2. Reducing diets—Popular works.
    3. Reducing exercises—Popular works.   I. Title: Eight minutes in the
morning for real shapes, real sizes.   II. Title.
    RM222.2.C77   2003
    613.7—dc21   2003001273

Distributed to the book trade by St. Martin's Press
2 4 6 8 10 9 7 5 3 1   hardcover

Visit us on the Web at www.rodalestore.com, or call us toll-free at (800) 848-4735.

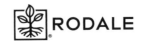

RODALE
WE INSPIRE AND ENABLE PEOPLE TO IMPROVE
THEIR LIVES AND THE WORLD AROUND THEM

Notice

The information given here is designed to help you make informed decisions about your body and health. The suggestions for specific foods, nutritional supplements, and exercises in this program are not intended to replace appropriate or necessary medical care. Before starting any exercise program, always see your physician. If you have specific medical symptoms, consult your physician immediately. If any recommendations given in this program contradict your physician's advice, be sure to consult your doctor before proceeding. Mention of specific products, companies, organizations, or authorities in this book does not imply endorsement by the author or the publisher, nor does mention of specific companies, organizations, or authorities in the book imply that they endorse the book. The author and the publisher disclaim any liability or loss, personal or otherwise, resulting from the procedures in this program. Internet addresses and telephone numbers given in this book were accurate at the time the book went to press.

To my beautiful wife, Heather.

Thank you for your support, inspiration, and unending love.

You are my best friend. I love you with all my heart, baby doll.

Acknowledgments

First, I want to thank my 3 million-and-growing weight-loss clients at JorgeCruise.com whom I have had the privilege of coaching. Without their feedback, insights, and support, *8 Minutes in the Morning for Real Shapes, Real Sizes* would not be the success it is today.

To Emme, the true role model for all "real shapes." Her message to love your body, no matter what size, is the heart of this book. Thanks, Emme, for being the inspiration, for being real, and for being above the curve. Bravo!

I must thank Oprah Winfrey, the lady who launched my career. She invited me to be a guest on her show in Chicago and introduced me to two people whose lives had changed because of my Web site. I will never forget that day. From that moment on, I knew that the Internet was a powerful resource that could change people's lives and bodies.

Heather, my wife, whom I love so much. Thanks again, baby doll, for being my muse.

Jan Miller, my literary agent, and Michael Broussard, her right arm, thank you for making *8 Minutes in the Morning* a reality and best-seller. I look forward to a lifetime of great weight-loss books with you.

Anthony Robbins and Pam Hendrickson, his right hand, thank you for your friendship, support, and inspiration. You are an extraordinary force for good in the world.

Dr. Andrew Weil and Michele Hardin, his right hand, thank you so much for empowering the world with your message of integrative medicine. You are a man who has changed my health and life. Thank you so much.

Mark Victor Hansen, thank you for your support and for being my role model on how to create a best-selling book. You are a gem.

Carol Brooks and Margaret Jaqua for your friendship and initial support. Thanks so much!

Dad, thank you for giving me a major boost when I was starting off. Your initial support helped me plant seeds that have grown to be strong and independent oak trees.

To my sister, Marta, for her love. To my *Abuelita* Maria (grandma) for her lifelong devotion. *Mil besitos.* And of course to my beautiful Mama, Gloria, and her many sacrifices that allow me to stand where I am today.

To Mike Sr., Mike Jr., Sue, and Kathy. Thanks for being part of my family and life. I love you guys.

To Lisa Sharkey, my friend who has a heart of gold.

To Bruce Barlean and the whole Barlean's family. Thanks for everything.

To my buddy and great friend, Jade Beutler, and his family.

To all my friends at Guthy-Renker and Schulberg Media.

To Katrina Goddard for her outstanding editorial support.

To the Rodale team and their immediate belief in *8 Minutes in the Morning for Real Shapes, Real Sizes.* In particular, I thank Alisa Bauman for helping me to stay on track and convey my message, Jennifer Kushnier for managing all the project details, Elizabeth Shimer for her stellar research skills, Chris Rhoads for designing a beautiful book, Jackie Dornblaser for getting me where I needed to go, Keith Biery for his layout wizardry, and Stephanie Tade, who truly made this project possible. Also a special thank you to Jim Gallucci, Kelly Schmidt, Dana Bacher, Marc Jaffe, Steve Murphy, and the Rodale family.

Thanks to Robert Trachtenberg for the excellent cover photo and to Mitch Mandel at Rodale for the interior photos. Great job!

And finally, to my extraordinary and magical public relations team: Cindy Ratzlaff at Rodale, Mary Lengle, and Arielle Ford and her team in San Diego. Thank you all so much from the bottom of my heart for your hard work, time, and efforts! Thank you, thank you, thank you!

Foreword

Did you know that 62 million American women wear a size 12 or larger? Unfortunately, we live in a society that puts a high priority on the unrealistic attainment of beauty, forcing men and women to yearn for a body size much smaller than ideal.

But things are changing! Through my lectures, television appearances, books, and women's advocacy projects, I've made it my mission to help children and adults understand that our self-esteem and personal happiness are not dependent upon our dress sizes or weight.

Jorge Cruise's *8 Minutes in the Morning for Real Shapes, Real Sizes* is also helping to lead this change. It's truly the first weight-loss plan that does not make thinness your goal. Rather, the plan challenges you to be the *best* you can be. Jorge has a big, bold, and beautiful message: Be who you are and be as healthy as possible while doing it.

When you follow his plan, you will get many positive results—and not just on a physical level. Jorge's message is about self-acceptance and health. Yes, he will help you lose the extra weight that might be slowing you down and holding you back. But that does not mean you must become a tiny size. Rather, you'll reach a realistic "real shape" for you and your body type. Yes, you will fit into a smaller pair of pants, but more important, you'll also feel healthier and achieve a higher quality of life.

Perhaps Jorge's most important lesson is that you must accept your body as it is today, regardless of your size. That is *his* life's mission and his first secret to becoming healthier and happier.

I wish you the best in your upcoming adventure with Jorge. Have a great time, and include your friends and family!

Emme

www.emmesupermodel.com

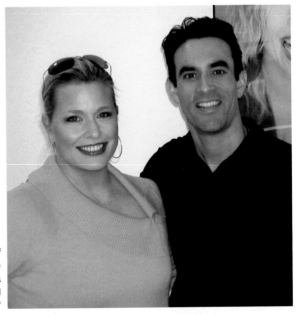

Emme is a full-figured supermodel, the television host of *Fashion Emergency* on E! Entertainment Television and the STYLE network, a best-selling author, a lecturer, and a clothing designer. No wonder *People* magazine selected her twice as one of the "50 Most Beautiful People."

Contents

Part 1: Jorge and You

Part 2: How It Works

Part 3: The Program

Part 4: Beyond the 8 Minutes

Introduction

I've struggled with extra weight for as long as I can remember. I've tried just about every weight-loss plan, including pills, shots, and various types of exercise equipment. Regardless of the method, I almost always lost weight. But without fail, I always gained it back (and then some).

Before Jorge's *8 Minutes in the Morning for Real Shapes, Real Sizes* plan, I thought I was too busy to eat breakfast. I survived on fast food. I always got it "supersized." Everything in my closet was black, fit loosely, and had elastic banding. I used clothing to hide my body.

Food provided instant gratification. I used it as a stress reliever. Many times when I was unhappy, I'd eat to make myself feel better. But then I'd feel sad because I knew I would only get heavier, so I'd eat some more and say, "What the heck. It doesn't matter anyway."

It all changed one day when I discovered Jorge Cruise's weight-loss program. At first, I didn't completely believe that I could lose weight while exercising only 8 minutes a day. However, with my busy schedule, I knew that 8 minutes was all I had. I decided to give it a try.

I saw and felt a difference within 2 weeks. Prior to starting on this life-changing journey, I frequently got headaches, felt sluggish, lacked energy and focus. Shortly after starting Jorge's program, my headaches stopped, my energy increased, and my cravings went away.

In 9 months, **I lost 70 pounds, averaging 2 pounds a week**. Since then, I've maintained my weight loss and have felt wonderful. I have lots of energy. I used to run from anyone who had a camera, but now I ask people to take my picture. I love the view I see when I catch my reflection in a mirror. I now have a new life. I feel and look different. I've changed my hair color and am looking forward to finding a significant other.

Why did Jorge's program work when so many others had failed? Well, it zeroed in on the source of my problem. Jorge taught me to break my addiction to food by establishing a loving and supporting network of close friends.

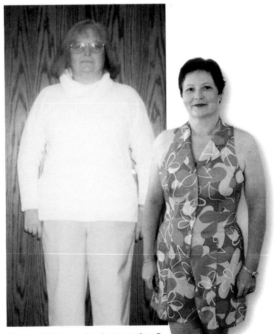

Doesn't Karen look amazing?
She's an 8-minute marvel who lost 70 pounds!

Jorge suggests that we have several support groups. We should have an accountability coach, a group of e-mail buddies, and several phone buddies. This support system not only helped me stay focused, it also helped to fill a void in my heart, the void that I had tried to fill with food.

No other program has ever given me this. No other program helps you deal with the source of the problem—the reason for overeating.

I'm just an ordinary person, just like you. There's nothing special about me. It only takes 8 minutes a day and a bit of planning in order to make the biggest change you'll ever experience. You say, "Not me?" I say, "Yes, you." Believe me, if I can do this program, you can do it, too!

—Karen Kraeszig

From the Desk of Jorge Cruise

Dear Friend,

Are you ready to start losing up to 2 pounds each week? I sure hope so. Congratulations on embarking on this incredible journey of transforming your body, health, and life! I respect you enormously. I believe we are kindred spirits on this path to constant never-ending health and happiness.

8 Minutes in the Morning for Real Shapes, Real Sizes will make your weight-loss experience simple and enjoyable. After my first *New York Times* best-selling weight-loss book, *8 Minutes in the Morning*, I received countless e-mails and letters asking me to create a specialized plan for the needs of busy, full-figured men and women who wanted to lose 30 or more pounds.

Voilà. *8 Minutes in the Morning for Real Shapes, Real Sizes* is the first weight-loss plan designed for the people who want to lose 30 *or more* pounds. What's the secret? Before learning my all-new, specialized 8-minute Cruise Moves, you will discover the following two critical secrets to end self-sabotage:

Secret 1: Accept yourself whatever your size.

Secret 2: Eliminate emotional eating by healing your hungry heart.

Then once you are emotionally fit, you will be ready to start burning 2 pounds each week with my brand-new Cruise Moves that require no equipment, no aerobics, and no trips to the gym. Add in my Cruise Down Plate eating system, and you will bring back the joy of eating without deprivation, starvation, or calorie counting. So get ready to improve your health and feel great about yourself in just 8 minutes a day!

Your friend,

JorgeCruise

America's #1 online weight-loss specialist

www.jorgecruise.com

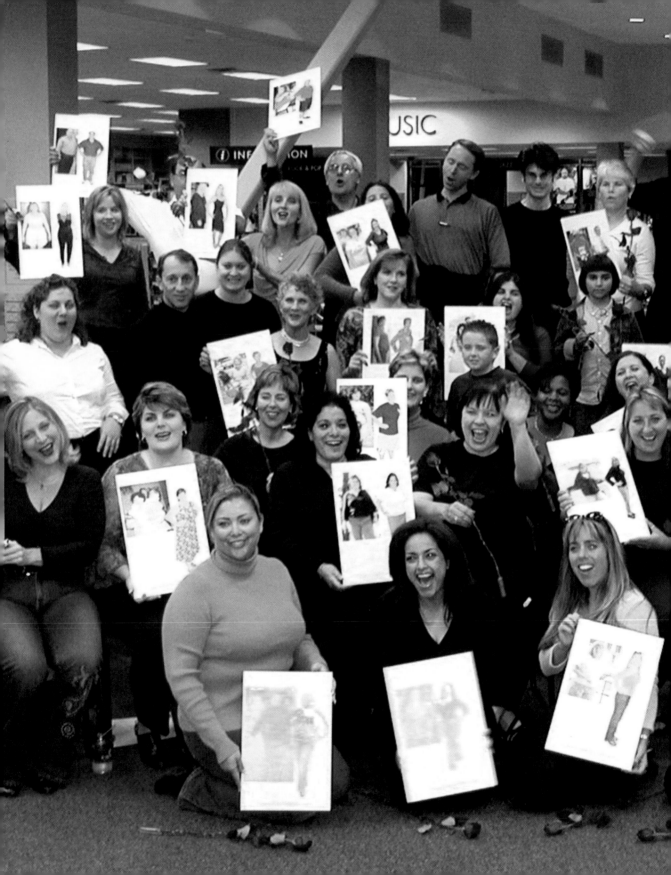

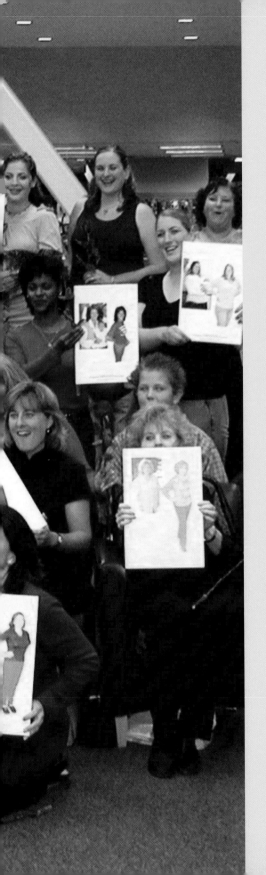

1
Jorge and You

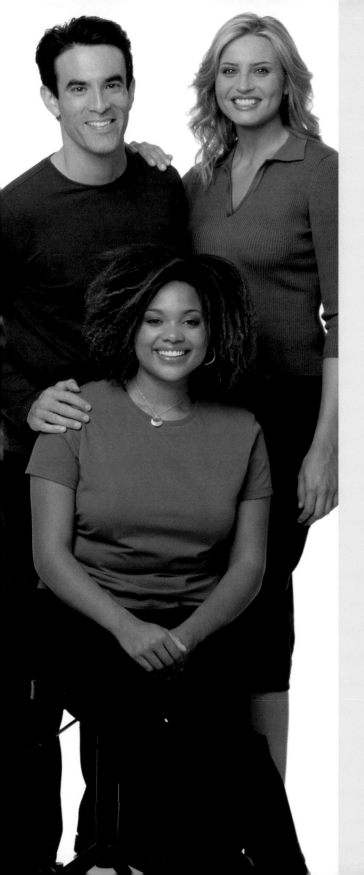

1
The Real Story

The Birth of
*8 Minutes in
the Morning for
Real Shapes,
Real Sizes*

a real program for real people

Are you short on time and have more than 30 pounds to lose? Frustrated with complicated, expensive, and time-consuming weight-loss programs that require you to count calories, starve and deprive yourself, buy expensive exercise equipment, go to the gym, or perform movements that hurt your knees or back? You've come to the right place. Welcome to the first weight-loss program specifically developed for busy people with real shapes and real sizes.

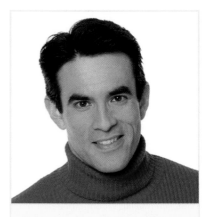

"I learned my most important lessons about weight-loss success from people just like you."

how it all began

It had been less than a month since I appeared on CNN and *Good Morning America*, and my JorgeCruise.com Web site was crazily abuzz. In those few weeks, membership to my site jumped from 3 million to 3.4 million Cruisers.

More than 450,000 people had joined my Web site in less than a month. I was amazed! Before I knew it, I received a call from my publisher, who told me that my first book, *8 Minutes in the Morning*, had hit the *New York Times* best-seller list.

I felt proud to know that my childhood struggles with weight and the related emotional pain—whether it was being picked on by other kids, not being able to keep up in gym class, or hearing myself referred to as "fatty butt"—had served a purpose. If it weren't for those initial struggles, I would never have dedicated my life to helping others lose weight and get healthy and happy.

So many people had e-mailed me, telling me how my program helped them to consistently shed 2 pounds each week. I read thousands of e-mails from people who had lost 5, 10, 15, 20, and 25 pounds with *8 Minutes in the Morning*.

They thanked me for a nutrition plan that allowed them to eat delicious foods, an exercise plan that took only 8 minutes to complete, and an overall program that was simple to follow. They loved being able to lose an average of 2 pounds each week in just 8 minutes a day. They were busy people, and they told me that this was the first weight-loss program that actually fit into their busy lives.

But I began to notice a defining trend to these e-mails and letters. Almost none of those who wrote to me had lost more than 30 pounds. I began to wonder why.

my awakening

I didn't have to wait long for the answer. A few e-mails and letters began to trickle in from people who wanted to lose *more than* 30 pounds. More and more similar e-mails and letters soon arrived. Then, it seemed everywhere I went—whether it was Indianapolis, Dallas, Seattle, Portland, Miami, Kentucky, St. Louis, New York City, San Diego, or Los Angeles—full-figured people began pulling me aside and telling me *their* stories, needs, and desires. They opened my eyes.

They would tell me, "Jorge, my sister bought your first book and has lost 15 pounds. She is very happy. But I have more than 30 to lose. I need your help because I can't do some of the

moves in your program. They are too advanced." Other men and women were making similar comments. Others wrote and told me that they became out of breath when trying to do my original *8 Minutes in the Morning* routines that required them to switch back and forth between laying, sitting, or standing. Some complained of knee or back discomfort with particular exercises. Others said using dumbbells was not practical for them when they traveled.

There it was, the answer to my question. It was as if someone had flipped on a light switch and I could finally see the reality. I realized my first weight-loss program simply didn't work well for people with more than 30 pounds to lose. At that moment, I realized that I had really developed an initial program for the average person who wanted to lose *less* than 30 pounds. For full-figured women or men, these exercises were too hard on the joints, particularly the knees.

It all came together one day when I picked up *USA Today* and read the following headline on the front page: "6 in 10 Are Overweight; Health Fallout Is Feared." The story went on to quote new statistics from the National Health and Nutrition Examination Survey,

inside facts

People with 30 pounds or more to lose need a realistic weight-loss plan that is about being healthy and *not about being skinny*. I challenge you to commit yourself *right now* to my *8 Minutes in the Morning for Real Shapes, Real Sizes* program for 4 weeks. After 4 weeks, I'm convinced you'll want to stick with the program for the rest of your life.

8 Minutes in the Morning for Real Shapes, Real Sizes will show you how to:

1. Consistently **lose up to 2 pounds each week** and improve your health

2. **Accept yourself** and your body no matter what your size

3. **Stop overeating** by filling yourself up with true nurturing and support rather than food

4. **Receive the undying support** from others just like you (online)

5. **Exercise comfortably**, no matter how large your body size

6. **Automatically eat the right amount of food**, without counting calories, fat grams, or food groups

statistics that placed a startling 65 percent of American adults in the overweight or obese category. The story quoted the same definition for obesity that I had seen years before when I studied weight control science and nutrition at the University of California at San Diego and when I studied biomechanics at the Cooper Institute in Dallas. It defined obesity as being 30 or more pounds heavier than a healthy body weight. *Bingo!* I got it. I knew what I had to do.

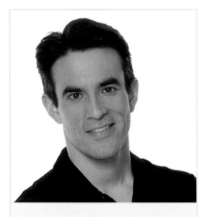

"As much as we hate body fat, all of us, particularly women, need some of it to survive."

designed just for you

I realized that millions of men and women needed a weight-loss program designed specifically for those with more than 30 pounds to lose. They needed a simple weight-loss program designed for real shapes and real sizes. That realization led to the creation of this book.

Welcome to the revolutionary weight-loss program designed for your body shape and size. It requires no exercise equipment, no aerobics, and no trips to the gym. I tested all of my Cruise Moves in *8 Minutes in the Morning for Real Shapes, Real Sizes* on people just like you. They work. They won't feel uncomfortable. You'll love them.

In addition to an exercise plan custom fit to your body, *8 Minutes in the Morning for Real Shapes, Real Sizes* also offers my special Cruise Down Plate eating system. It's an extremely simple and delicious system that will help you shed pounds. The Cruise Down Plate will bring back the joy of eating without calorie counting, deprivation, or starvation dieting. You'll be able to eat all the foods you love—and still lose weight!

But it doesn't stop there. I've learned from my millions of clients that the best eating and exercise program in the world will never work unless you first make a change deep inside, a change that will help you to effortlessly fuel your motivation for weight loss. This deep inner change is so crucial that I've spent two entire chapters of this book—chapters 2 and 3—laying out the framework needed for you to make it happen. Once you flip this deep inner switch, you'll literally train your brain for weight loss.

So get ready to lose 30 or more pounds once and for all. You'll feel fantastic in just 8 minutes a day! I hope you're as excited as I am about this program. I know you'll love it.

my background

Well, believe it or not, I haven't always looked like the photo of myself on the cover of this book. Just look at the picture of me on this page, and you'll see what I looked like as a kid. At that time, I was traveling quickly down the road to an unhealthy life. I'm convinced I would easily weigh well over 300 pounds today if I had not changed my eating patterns and lifestyle.

my full family

So, you see, I know what it's like to feel embarrassed about extra weight. I've been there. And so has my dad, my sister, my grandfather, and my grandmother. We were a family of large people, that's for sure.

I grew up in Southern California in a Mexican-American home. My mom was from Mexico and my dad from Pennsylvania. Both sides of my family loved to eat huge food portions. In our home, food and love were woven together as tightly as a silk cocoon. Because my mom loved me so much, guess what she did? She fed me big portions.

And because I loved my mom, I wanted to make her happy, so I ate everything she fed me. My mom's mom, *Abuelita* Maria, also lived with us. And, of course, she loved me, too. My mom would feed me one meal,

and before I knew it, my *abuelita* (*grandma* in Spanish) would feed me another. I consumed enormous quesadillas, bologna sandwiches, and nachos. If I didn't eat everything on my plate, mom or grandmom took it very personally. I soon lost touch with my true hunger and began to eat not as a way to fill my belly, but rather, as a way to fill my heart and my soul.

By age 10, I was a roly-poly kid. My mom began calling me *el rey*, which in Spanish means "the king."

I was also extremely unfit. My family believed that exercise was hard and time-consuming. My mom and dad were busy, working 10-

hour days. We *never* moved or exercised as a family. I can't remember ever playing football, basketball, or baseball with my dad. I have no memories of doing anything active with him or my mom.

As I grew older, the lack of exercise and excess food began to take its toll. By the time I was 15, I had severe asthma, very little energy, and daily headaches. My extra weight hurt me the most at school, where the kids teased me and called me names. I was that kid who was always picked last

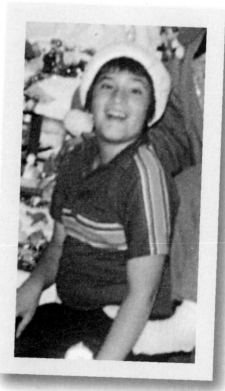

At age 10, I was already chubby. The kids at school called me "fatty butt."

on any sports team. One day in gym class, the teacher asked us to do a number of push-ups. I couldn't even complete one. I felt embarrassed, and the other children teased me. I began to feel like a reject, a nothing.

But I wasn't the only one in my family who was suffering from body size.

my dad teaches us all a lesson

When I was 18, my dad, who until then had had a big belly for as long as I could remember, was diagnosed with prostate cancer. The doctors gave him 1 year to live, with no medical intervention, and from 5 to 6 years with prostate surgery, chemotherapy, and radiation.

The death sentence scared my

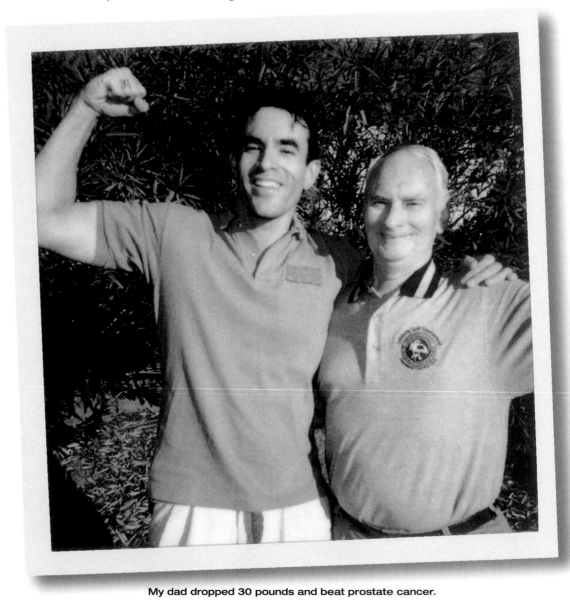

My dad dropped 30 pounds and beat prostate cancer.

dad much less than the implications. He knew that surgery would probably render him incontinent and impotent. He decided to forgo medical intervention—a decision that not only changed his life but also the lives of everyone in his family, including mine.

Instead of opting for surgery, my dad enrolled in an alternative health center in San Diego. I was so shaken by my dad's diagnosis, I checked into the center, too. We learned about nutrition, particularly about fiber, whole grains, fruits, and vegetables.

Dad and I completely overhauled our diets. We began drinking more water, eating more vegetables, and reducing our food portions. One day I realized that my headaches and asthma symptoms were gone, and my energy levels had improved.

Dad's recovery was much more dramatic. He lost 30 pounds. Remember that 1-year death sentence? Well, that was more than 14 years ago, and dad is still going strong!

dorothy, my big, bold, and beautiful grandmother

A year later, during a summer break from Dartmouth College in New Hampshire, I visited my dad's parents who lived in Altoona, Pennsylvania. I had not

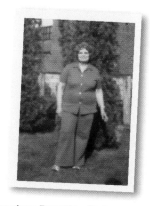

Grandma Dorothy died as a result of her excess weight.

seen them in a few years and couldn't wait to get to know them better. During that break, I spent a lot of time with my big, bold, and beautiful grandmother, Dorothy. She was a very loving soul.

All her life she was a big lady who loved to eat and hated to exercise.

She was just like me. Food was her friend, and exercise was time-consuming and hard on her joints. I do have to say that she did go to the mall with my grandpa for about an hour once a week to do a little walking and a little window-shopping. She looked forward to it every week. Unfortunately, these trips never did help her lose much weight.

After spending time with her during that summer break, I could see that it was getting very difficult for her to walk up stairs and to even walk at the mall. At 5

foot 4, she weighed almost 200 pounds and had high blood pressure and high cholesterol.

She did not think much of it, until she had her first stroke. After that stroke, she and my grandpa decided to move to San Diego to be closer to my dad. Unfortunately, it was too late for my grandma. Shortly after they arrived, she suffered a second stroke and passed away.

my sister accepts and wins

If you read my first book, you also met my wonderful and gorgeous sister, Marta, who lost more than 40 pounds. But I didn't tell you then that the real secret to her success was learning to accept herself, no matter what her size. She, like many of us, got hypnotized into thinking that she had to be skinny and a size 0 or 2 to be healthy.

That's just not true. In fact, a size 2 or 0 may actually be as unhealthy as a size 30. As much as we hate body fat, all of us, particularly women, need some of it to survive. You see, fat cells secrete a hormone called leptin. Among other things, leptin tells your brain whether your body has enough stored calories (a.k.a. body fat) to support the growth, delivery, and feeding of a baby. When your brain senses that leptin levels are too low, it responds by shutting down your reproductive cycle.

Ladies, I know some of you might be thinking, "Yay! No more menstrual cycle." But before you start looking forward to this, you must know that lack of menstruation is not normal. When your brain shuts down your reproductive cycle, it also lowers the female hormone estrogen. This is the same hormone that helps to protect you against bone loss and heart disease and gives you your womanly shape.

Numerous studies show that superthin athletes, models, and people with anorexia tend to suffer from abnormally low bone mineral density and advanced stages of heart disease. And reports from Hollywood personal trainers, nutritionists, and other insiders reveal that the increasing number of actresses who weigh less than 100 pounds and stand more than 5 feet 5 inches tall achieve their unnaturally thin looks in unhealthy ways.

Armed with those facts, I helped my sister discover that, though thin might be in, thin certainly is *not* normal or healthy. In fact, the average American woman is a size 12 or 14, *not* a size 2 to 6.

Once Marta understood this fact, she stopped aspiring to look like superthin models or actresses and instead began aspiring to look like normal-sized women, women with realistic body shapes and sizes, women who wear a size 12 or larger. (You'll learn how to do the same in chapter 2.) She chose role models such as supermodel Emme, actress Delta Burke, singer Queen Latifah, and models Mia Tyler, Carré Otis, and Kate Dillon, real women who look great—even if they aren't a size 6—and who are healthy!

Once Marta accepted that she may *never* look as thin as a supermodel (who spends all day at a gym and probably subsists on carrot sticks), she was able to find the motivation to stick to a weight-loss program. Today she's

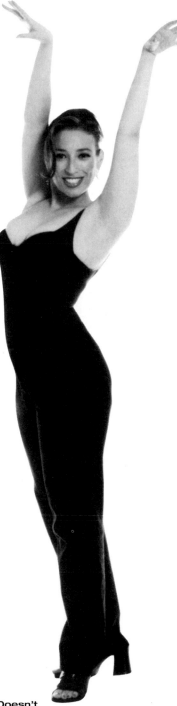

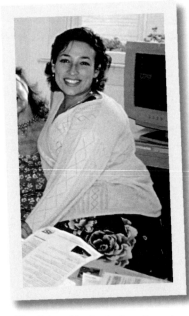

My sister, Marta, before learning to accept her body.

Marta today. Doesn't she look fantastic?

lost more than 40 pounds. She's a size 12, and she looks and feels fantastic.

So you see, over the years, I've learned many important lessons about weight-loss success through my personal experiences as well as those of my family members. I've also learned quite a bit by studying weight control and nutrition at UC-San Diego and the Cooper Institute. But I probably learned my most important lessons about weight loss from people just like you.

thousands of e-mails

As I already shared with you, I received countless e-mails and letters from busy, full-figured women and men who begged me to adapt the exercises from *8 Minutes in the Morning* to their fuller bodies. They told me that these original exercises were too advanced. They told me that they wanted an even simpler program, one that required absolutely no equipment—not even dumbbells. They wanted a program that they could do *anywhere*.

Erin McLeod was one of those people. When she first wrote to me, she weighed 75 pounds more than her healthy weight. She's a single mother with two children, attends college full-time, and holds down a part-time job as a

bartender. "There is just not a lot of time left for me," she told me. "Some days I am so busy that I can't even fit a shower into my schedule!"

Can you relate to that?

Erin is just one of hundreds of people who inspired me to design *8 Minutes in the Morning for Real Shapes, Real Sizes*. (Read her story and see her before and after photos on page 12.) Feedback from Erin and others made me realize that I needed to write another book, one for the millions of people with real shapes and real sizes, for the millions of busy people who wanted to lose much more than 30 pounds. I realized that I had to write the prequel to my first book, one that would help people lose enough weight and get in enough shape to move on to the original *8 Minutes in the Morning* program.

Unfortunately, I now realize that I should have written this book first.

I wasted no time. I busily went to work to create a specialized and exclusive *8 Minutes in the Morning* plan for my larger clients. I tested exercise after exercise, food plan after food plan, and motivational concept after motivational concept on thousands of clients—online, over the telephone, and in person. Erin, who lives in San Diego, was one of those testers.

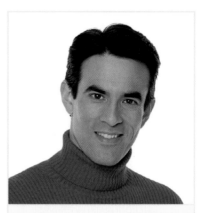

"Two pounds is the average amount of fat you can lose in a week. This will allow your skin to properly recoil and thus avoid sagging and wrinkles."

I'll admit, writing this book and designing this program wasn't always easy. I didn't get it right on the first try, or even the second, or the third. More than 10,000 people tested the entire program more than once, telling

erin mcleod lost 75 pounds

Before I started Jorge's plan, I had gone from desperate to hopeless. I was so fat that I hated to go out in public and couldn't play with my kids.

"I now take my kids to the beach and the park, and we run and play and have a great time."

My family and coworkers have all commented on my success. My ex-husband even told me that I look great!

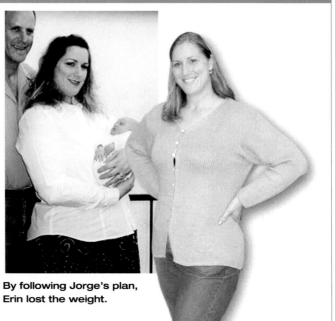

By following Jorge's plan, Erin lost the weight.

me over and over what worked and what did not.

Finally, I got it right. I am thrilled to tell you that the book you hold in your hands contains everything you need to lose 30 or more pounds in the easiest manner ever. You will truly love it.

Erin sure did. These days she's out of bed by 6 A.M. She does her 8 minutes of moves first thing, while her kids are asleep. Then she drinks a pint of water, eats breakfast, and has even found the time to relax and watch the news for 10 minutes before waking her kids up at 7 o'clock.

"Every morning, my two-year-old wakes up and says to me, 'Mom, you are the best.' Now I feel like I deserve his praise," she told me after losing 75 pounds with the program. "The quality of time I share with my children has improved a thousand times since I started *8 Minutes in the Morning*. My energy level is so much higher. I feel better now than I have in years. I don't want to sound like a cliché, but if I can do this, anyone can!"

As Erin's story shows, *8 Minutes in the Morning for Real Shapes, Real Sizes* is the only weight-loss book that specifically addresses the needs of busy people will fuller figures.

When you embark on this journey, you will:

• Learn to accept yourself and your body, no matter what your size

• Replace emotional eating with a smarter method that allows you to experience the ultimate sense of support and comfort—without food

• Consistently lose up to 2 pounds a week

• Transform your life and feel fulfilled, whole, and happy

Follow *8 Minutes in the Morning for Real Shapes, Real Sizes*, and you will see amazing results in just 28 days.

why fat is not your fault

Earlier I mentioned my sister's story, how she couldn't find the motivation to stick to a weight-loss program until she first found realistic role models and chose a realistic goal. She couldn't succeed until she first fixed the source of her problem. She needed to first work on her internal demons, the ones that were telling her that she wasn't good enough, before she could find the energy reserve she needed to lose the weight for good.

Marta needed to walk away from the concept of losing weight to *look* better and embrace the concept of losing weight to *feel* better. Most people try to lose weight as a form of body punishment. After seeing image after image of superthin actors, actresses, and models, this is understandable.

As I mentioned earlier, many Hollywood actresses and actors are abnormally thin, and they achieve this superthinness in many unnatural and unhealthy ways. According to surveys, the models for *Playboy* centerfolds have been getting smaller since 1959, and since 1980, 99 percent of them have been underweight. One study found that 25 percent of them meet the criteria for anorexia. Researchers have also suggested that some of the most popular Hollywood actresses meet the criteria for anorexia. Finally, scientists also speculate that if most clothing store mannequins were actual human beings, they wouldn't menstruate.

One study in particular powerfully shows just how much the media influences the way we feel about our bodies. It looked at the differences in body dissatisfaction and eating attitudes in visually impaired women—women who could not be influenced by superthin media images because they could not *see* them. The re-

THE CONSEQUENCES OF EXCESS WEIGHT

Though many of us worry about the visual consequences of excess weight, the true dangers are to your health, longevity, and overall well-being.

- Being overweight and obese doubles your risk for heart failure.

- Just 22 extra pounds in a man makes him 75 percent more likely to have a heart attack.

- A weight gain of just 11 to 18 pounds doubles your risk of developing diabetes.

- Excess weight increases your risk for more than 25 diseases and conditions, including high blood pressure, gallbladder disease, kidney disease, liver disease, asthma, back pain, depression, chronic pain, and impaired immunity.

- According to the Centers for Disease Control and Prevention, more than 300,000 Americans die each year from weight-related illnesses, second only to tobacco-related deaths. Each *day*, more than 800 Americans die from complications of excess weight.

- You need to lose only a small fraction of that weight to dramatically improve your health. You need to lose only 5 to 10 percent of your weight to reduce blood pressure, cholesterol, and arthritis discomfort and to improve your blood sugar control.

FALSE CLAIMS
HAVE MISLED US ALL

As our waistlines and body sizes have increased over the years, a number of people and companies have tried to capitalize on our fears and body dissatisfaction by marketing weight-loss products with grossly exaggerated claims.

A Federal Trade Commission review of 300 weight-loss ads for 218 dietary supplements, diet patches, creams, wraps, and other products found that 40 percent of the ads made at least one false claim and 55 percent made a deceptive claim that could not be substantiated.

The deceptive claims included:

• "You could lose 8 to 10 pounds per week, easily . . . and you won't gain the weight back afterwards."

• "You can eat as much as 4,000 calories a day and still lose weight."

• "The only supplement that has been proven to increase fat loss 38.8 times more than diet or exercise alone."

• "Curbs cravings . . . reduces calorie absorption."

• "Lose 10 pounds in 48 hours. . . . Guaranteed."

They have misled us all into expecting fast, significant results without lifting a finger. Here's the bottom line: You can achieve simple and effective weight loss with *8 Minutes in the Morning for Real Shapes, Real Sizes*, but there is no miracle pill.

searchers found that women who had been blind since birth were much less dissatisfied with their bodies than women who had lost their sight later in life. Sighted women had the highest levels of body dissatisfaction and the most negative attitudes toward food!

So, you see, you are surrounded by images that trick you into thinking that you are not good enough, that hurt you so deeply inside that they destroy your motivation to stick to a program.

At the same time you are being bombarded with these body-image-damaging symbols, you're also being bombarded with marketing messages that encourage you to overeat. For example, it costs fast food restaurants very little to supersize your meal. They spend the majority of their revenue on labor, packaging, and marketing. To a fast food chain, supersize french fries actually cost them the same amount of revenue as small fries.

So they push the big portions in order to make you feel as if you're getting a bargain. The large fries may only cost you a few cents more than the small, but they add a huge wallop to your waistline. For example, a regular hamburger, fries, and

12-ounce soda used to amount to a reasonable 590 calories. The chain now advertises its supersize "Extra Value" meal with a Quarter Pounder with Cheese, supersize fries, and supersize soda for a total of 1,550 calories!

Fast food restaurants aren't the only establishments that are dishing up more food. Restaurant portions have also increased. And studies show, when we *see* more food, we tend to *eat* more food, regardless of our true calorie needs.

End result: We've become a fatter nation. While the average

weight of a Hollywood actress has dipped below 110 pounds and the average dress size below a size 4, the real, everyday woman has grown an inch larger than only 10 years ago, bringing the average dress size for real women to a size 14.

According to the Centers for Disease Control and Prevention, more than 64 percent of U.S. adults now weigh 30 or more pounds beyond a healthy weight. That totals more than 97 million people!

I tell all of my clients that nothing feels as good as knowing that you took charge of your life and changed your body. It's the difference between knowing you earned a trophy for your accomplishments or just going out and buying a trophy without actually earning it. You'd only feel proud about the trophy you earned. Weight loss is the same. Once you—not a pill or patch or cream—take control of your weight, you will feel terrific. That's a real success.

the power of acceptance

By following the plan in this book, you can lose a realistic and healthy 2 pounds a week. That's the average amount of fat you can lose in a week—healthfully. Some of you might lose more the first week or two. On average, however, you will lose what doctors deem safe, effective, and realistic—2 pounds a week.

realistic goals for real sizes

That's 8 pounds in 28 days. If you want to lose 30 pounds, it will take you 15 weeks to take off the weight. If you want to lose 60 pounds, it will take you 30 weeks. *8 Minutes in the Morning for Real Shapes, Real Sizes* will help you lose a realistic amount of weight, bringing you to a *realistic size*, and do so with a *realistic amount of exercise* and by eating *realistic food portions*.

When you embark on the *8 Minutes in the Morning for Real Shapes, Real Sizes* journey, you will lose 2 pounds a week by exercising and following a realistic—and simple—eating plan.

End result: You will reach a realistic weight for your body. Most important, you will keep that weight off for good. No more yo-yo dieting. You will lose that excess fat once and for all—and you'll feel fantastic as you do.

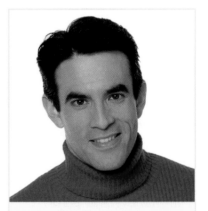

"Remember, losing 2 pounds a week ensures that skin recoils and doesn't sag."

your questions

How do I know if I'm overweight?

According to the Centers for Disease Control and Prevention, you're officially overweight when you weigh more than 30 pounds above your "healthy" weight. You will determine your healthy weight in chapter 3 on page 45.

the secret ingredients

Remember earlier when I told you that my program would teach you about a deep inner switch that would help fuel your motivation to lose weight? Well, here's the secret: body acceptance and nurturing. This is the most important ingredient to your success and what truly sets *8 Minutes in the Morning for Real Shapes, Real Sizes* apart from other weight-loss programs.

You see, one of the most important lessons that I've learned since writing my last book is that some of my clients were turning to food to lift their spirits, drown their sorrows, soothe their stress, and even calm their fears. Food had become their closest friend.

I realized I needed to create a concrete plan to help my clients reduce their dependence on food as a source of comfort. So I developed a two-step plan, outlined in chapters 2 and 3, to help them overcome emotional eating.

In chapter 2, you'll learn how body acceptance can fuel your weight loss. You see, study after study shows that positive body image provides the spark to eating healthfully and sticking to an exercise program. Body acceptance boosts your self-esteem, which in turn destroys self-destructive thought and eating patterns—which in turn helps you naturally gravitate to your realistic weight. This is the most important key to your success. Once you accept and nurture your body, your nutrition and exercise efforts will literally become effortless.

In chapter 3, you'll learn one more secret to help you heal your hungry heart and put an end to emotional eating. This secret lies in what I call The People Solution. The source of your problem lies deep inside. You must reach inside yourself to change your outer appearance.

Only when you are emotionally fit will you be ready to start using my revolutionary Cruise Moves and Cruise Down Plate eating system. So before you start the eating and exercise programs, you must complete all of the exercises in chapters 2 and 3. You must accept your body, heal your hungry heart, and enact The People Solution. You'll learn more about this exciting program soon, but first, let's take a look at the overall structure of *8 Minutes in the Morning for Real Shapes, Real Sizes*.

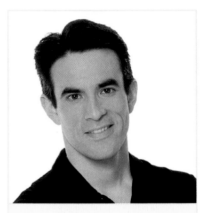

"Once you accept and nurture your body, your nutrition and exercise efforts will literally become effortless."

about the program

8 Minutes in the Morning for Real Shapes, Real Sizes will give you the tools you need to stay healthy for the rest of your life. Here's how it works. Each morning you will work on three things: your emotional success, your physical fitness success, and your eating success.

before the 8 minutes: your emotional success

Each day before your 8-minute exercise routine, I will help you get emotionally strong and fit. You will accomplish this with what I call The People Solution. This system—outlined in chapters 2 and 3 and expanded in chapter 7—will give you the advantage you need to move beyond self-sabotaging thinking and motivate yourself to love your new, fit lifestyle.

You may feel tempted to skip your daily People Solution exercises. Please don't! They are critical to your success. These daily

critical secrets

secret 1: Accept yourself whatever your size
secret 2: Heal your hungry heart

secrets will help you to fix yourself from the inside out, zeroing in on the source of your problem deep inside. They will help you to fully accept your body and nurture your heart and soul, helping you to flip an inner switch that will help you to naturally stop overeating and start exercising. They are the keys to your success.

the 8 minutes: your physical fitness success

My all-new Cruise Moves are the center of this program. They take only 8 minutes a day and require absolutely no equipment—not even dumbbells. You can do these moves anywhere. You don't need a gym membership. You don't need to buy anything. The only props you'll ever need—a wall, a chair, a table, a phone book—are already in your house.

No matter what your size, you will love these moves. Each morning, I will give you two new strength-training moves specifically designed to help you speed up your metabolism. I tested these moves on clients just like you, so I *know* you can do them. They are designed so that they will not hurt your back or knees. Not one move will make you feel off balance. Not one will make you feel like a failure.

Rather, my moves will help you firm up your body and burn fat as efficiently as possible. Each Sunday you'll take the day off. You'll learn more about why Cruise Moves are so effective in chapter 4. In chapter 5, you'll learn why I strongly suggest you do your Cruise Moves *in the morning*.

after the 8 minutes: your eating success

The Cruise Down Plate, which you'll read more about in chapters 6 and 10, is my latest secret that makes eating healthfully extremely easy—without counting any calories. Plus, it will never leave you feeling hungry or deprived again!

The Cruise Down Plate will teach you to fill up on low-calorie, delicious foods, how to use the right amount of fat to lower your appetite, and how to eat the right types of foods in the right portions—automatically.

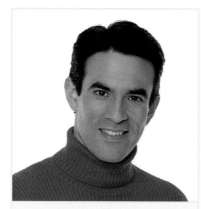

"I know what it's like to feel embarrassed about extra weight. I've been there."

There are no forbidden foods on the Cruise Down Plate. In fact, I suggest you eat a yummy treat every day. Get ready to bring back the real joy of eating!

So there you have it. The three elements of the program that you will tackle. But it doesn't stop there.

your recipe for success

Right now, I want you to find a quiet place to read chapters 2 and 3 without interruption. Why? Before you learn my specialized 8-minute moves, you must first accept yourself whatever your size, and you must heal your hungry heart. These are the two most critical secrets to real weight loss.

Chapters 2 and 3 will give you the essential foundation you require. Think of *8 Minutes in the Morning for Real Shapes, Real Sizes* as a recipe. If you were baking a cake, you wouldn't carelessly omit the baking powder or the flour or the sugar. If you did,

the cake might not rise or taste all that great.

It's the same with *8 Minutes in the Morning for Real Shapes, Real Sizes*. If you decide to skip any element of the program, you might not end up with the best results. Just as the baking powder and sugar are essential to the success of baking a cake, so is each aspect of this program. For example, if you skip your homework in chapters 2 and 3 and proceed directly to the program, I can't be certain you will lose weight. Similarly, if you do just one exercise a day rather than two, you may not achieve the best results.

You must include all of the suggested ingredients in the right order to experience fantastic results. So please, commit yourself right now to following every aspect of the program to your fullest potential.

In return, *8 Minutes in the Morning for Real Shapes, Real Sizes* will change your life. So get ready to get to it!

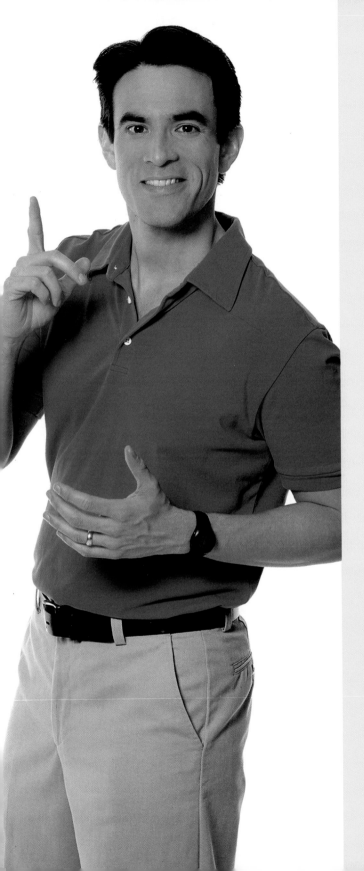

2
The First Secret to Weight-Loss Success

Accept, Respect, and Love Your Body Whatever Your Size

acceptance, respect, and love

In chapter 1, I told you a story about my sister, Marta—how she had tried and tried to stick to a weight-loss plan many times but didn't succeed until she learned to accept and respect herself and her body and then aim for a realistic weight.

inner change equals outer change

Countless numbers of clients have told me that the same held true for them. No matter how simple the weight-loss program, they couldn't seem to find the motivation to stick with it until they first made a change deep inside, a change that affected their entire outlook on weight loss.

Anne Armstrong was one of those clients. She hated her body. When you hate something, how do you treat it? Think about it. Well, in Anne's case, she ignored it.

"My body and I didn't get along," she told me in retrospect. "I didn't accept it. In fact, I hated the way it fit in clothes. I hated

the way it looked. I hated the image that stared back at me every time I looked in the mirror. I hated it so much that I ignored it completely. I focused all of my attention on other things, mostly work."

Anne worked such long hours that she never ate true meals. Her food life revolved around two food groups: the candy she ate at her desk and the fast food she ate during her commute. As a result, her weight became out of control. At her heaviest, she weighed 222 pounds.

When Anne came to me for help, I told her about the power of acceptance. I told her that she needed to stop hating her body and instead learn to treat it with love and respect. Once she learned this important secret to

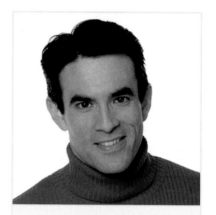

"Your body is an extraordinary machine that does extraordinary tasks every day."

weight-loss success, she lost 32 pounds! And the weight is still coming off.

"The moment I unconditionally accepted my body, I began to feel free," she said. "I began to treat my body with more honesty and respect. The moment I accepted my body for what it was, I felt a huge weight lift from my shoulders, and my life became mine and not a lie." (Read more about Anne below.)

Now, I want to teach you the secret that helped Anne, Marta, and countless others finally lose weight and keep it off. It's going to sound deceivingly simple, but here it is: *You must unconditionally and completely accept and respect your current body—right now—no matter how many pounds you wish to lose.*

I say that this is deceivingly simple because most people believe one of two falsehoods that prevent them from turning this secret into a reality:

1. They think they will accept and respect their bodies once they lose the weight they want to lose.

2. They think they already accept and respect their bodies.

Before you turn to the next chapter, you'll understand why both of those beliefs are false. For now, trust me on this. If you don't fully accept and respect your current body, you will never treat it as the most precious gift that has ever been given to you. If you don't respect your body and treat it as a precious gift, then you will never find the willpower and motivation to exercise each day, stick to healthy food portions, drink plenty of water, and get enough sleep.

That's why your first step in the *8 Minutes in the Morning for Real Shapes, Real Sizes* plan will be to discover how to deeply and wholeheartedly feel that you are "good enough" and "amazing enough" *right now*—no matter how much weight you want to lose. Are you ready to take that step? Let's get started!

anne armstrong lost 32 pounds

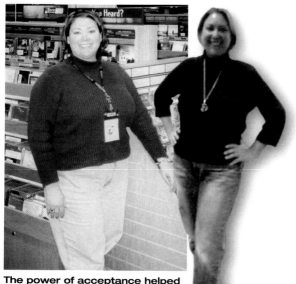

The power of acceptance helped Anne drop the pounds.

Before I started Jorge's plan, I was fat and frumpy. I didn't feel attractive. Men didn't want to meet me.

"Now, when I go out, I'm noticed."

I have also spied some of my male friends doing a double take when I walk into a room. I have been invited to more functions. I have lost my fear of being photographed and interviewed, and I love going out with the girls once again.

the power of unconditional acceptance

Let's start with the first myth I mentioned earlier. You must accept and respect your body right now—not once you lose the weight.

Many people falsely think that they will instantly begin to love their bodies once they lose the weight they feel they need to lose. That's simply not true. I know this because some of the most tortured people I've ever met have also been some of the thinnest. Ask just about any person from a size 6 to a size 26 about their weight-loss needs,

your "8 minute" edge

If you accept and respect your body:

• Your health will consistently become your number one priority

• You will effortlessly make the best decisions for your body

• You will learn the most important secret to finally shedding the pounds and keeping them off forever

• You will unlock your deepest and most powerful motivation to exercise and eat healthy portions

and most will tell you that they really need to lose a few pounds. They'll call their bodies nasty names that they wouldn't call their worst enemies.

Still not convinced? Well, a *Glamour* magazine survey found that 61 percent of respondents were ashamed of their hips, 64 percent of their stomachs, and 72 percent of their thighs—regardless of their current body size. Studies further show that 30 percent of women aspire to attain a body size that's 20 percent underweight, and 44 percent aspire to a size that's 10 percent underweight.

So, if you think that a smaller body size will automatically result in better body acceptance, you've put the cart before the horse. Rather, body acceptance will result in a smaller body size—not the other way around. Once you learn to accept and respect your body, you will instantly treat it differently.

Let me give you an example. Imagine you just bought yourself something expensive, something you've wanted for a long time and worked hard to earn. For example, let's say you just bought a brand new, ultra-expensive BMW convertible.

How would you treat it?

You'd treat it carefully, right? You'd drive off the car lot nice and slow. You'd certainly look

both ways as you pulled onto the road. You'd stay an extra-safe distance behind the car in front of you—no tailgating today! And you'd be hyperaware of every other car on the road.

You'd park far away from other cars in parking lots. You'd fill the car with premium gasoline. You'd faithfully change the oil every 3,000 miles. You'd park it in the garage instead of leaving it out in the rain. You'd routinely wash off every smudge. You'd never eat fast food while you were driving, and you certainly wouldn't let your teenage son drive it to school!

Am I right? That's certainly how I would treat a brand-new, expensive car.

Now let's take a look at the opposite scenario. How would you treat an older, "not-so-nice" car? Let's say the car's paint had rusted off a long time ago. Maybe the seats have faded and become threadbare. There are already a few stains on the floor and maybe even a few dents in the bumper.

Would you drive this car extra slow on the highway? Would you take care not to tailgate? Would you park it far away from other cars at the strip mall? Would you wash and wax it every week? Would you tune it up? Would you change the oil every 3,000 miles?

THE VALUE OF HEALTH

Whenever you need a little inspiration to put your body *first*, read over this list of powerful quotes from business leaders, historical figures, and some of the greatest thinkers of all time.

"A wise man should consider that health is the greatest of human blessings, and learn how by his own thought to derive benefit from his illnesses."

—Hippocrates (460 BC–377 BC)

"Health is not valued till sickness comes."

—Thomas Fuller, 1732

"It is health that is real wealth and not pieces of gold and silver."

—Gandhi

"What is called genius is the abundance of life and health."

—Henry David Thoreau

"Health is worth more than learning."

—Thomas Jefferson (1743–1826), letter to his cousin John Garland Jefferson, June 11, 1790

"The first wealth is health."

—Ralph Waldo Emerson

"True friendship is like sound health; the value of it is seldom known until it is lost."

—Charles Caleb Colton

"Those who do not find time for exercise will have to find time for illness."

—Earl of Derby

"Wisdom is to the mind what health is to the body."

—Francois De La Rochefoucauld

"A man or woman too busy to take care of his health is like a mechanic too busy to take care of his tools."

—Spanish proverb

"Imagine life as a game in which you are juggling five balls in the air. You name them—work, family, health, friends, and spirit—and you're keeping all of these in the air. You will soon understand that work is a rubber ball. If you drop it, it will bounce back. But the other four balls—family, health, friends, and spirit—are made of glass. If you drop one of these, they will be irrevocably scuffed, marked, nicked, damaged, or even shattered. They will never be the same. You must understand that and strive for balance in your life."

—Brian Dyson, CEO of Coca-Cola Enterprises from 1959–1994

"He who has health has hope; and he who has hope has everything."

—Arabian proverb

"When health is absent, wisdom cannot reveal itself, art cannot manifest, strength cannot fight, wealth becomes useless, and intelligence cannot be applied."

—Herophilus

"Ill health, of body or of mind, is defeat. Health alone is victory. Let all men, if they can manage it, contrive to be healthy!"

—Thomas Carlyle

lenora hennessy lost 42 pounds

Before I met Jorge Cruise, I was existing, but not living. My health and body were not a priority to me. As a result, my right knee was giving out, the bottoms of my feet felt bruised, and I was experiencing heart palpitations.

"Once I made my health and my body my first priority, everything changed."

Now that I have lost 42 pounds, I am now getting a lot of opposite-sex attention— yee-haw! I'm sassy and 17 again—body, mind, and spirit. I now realize that I am on the right track and have an incredible and bright new future ahead of me.

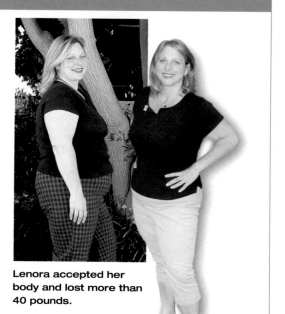

Lenora accepted her body and lost more than 40 pounds.

I doubt it. Yes, you'd neglect this car. What would happen before long? Would that car get better, stay the same, or fall apart more quickly? You know the answer.

But now imagine what would happen if, instead of neglecting that old car, you began treating it like that brand-new BMW. What if you started changing the oil, taking it in for tune-ups, washing and waxing it regularly, and telling your teenage son to keep his hands off?

It would become a nicer car. Suddenly the old paint job would start to shine, and the car would start to run like its old self. You'd proudly tell your friends, "Yes,

it's still running great after all these years."

Your body is a lot like that old car. If you begin to fill it with the best foods, slowly ease it onto the highway of fitness, and prevent yourself and others from inflicting nicks and dents with verbal abuse, it will respond by performing better than you ever dreamed.

Even better, your body will outperform that old car. If you accept, respect, and love your current body, it will transform itself not just into a better or nicer body, but rather into a brand-new body. No car can do that— only the precious human body can. No matter what age, or how

overweight, it is, the human body can transform itself into something that's healthier and stronger—with your help, of course.

Here's the best benefit of truly respecting your current body without any conditions: You will consistently ensure that *you* are your highest priority in your life. Work, the kids, your spouse, the phone, television, e-mail, and everything else will come second.

How do I know this is true? I have worked with more than 3 million clients. I know from my most successful 8-minute marvels that real weight loss only happens once your body becomes your highest priority. It's that simple.

If you don't respect your body, you'll place lots of other priorities ahead of your body's needs. When it's time to exercise in the morning, you'll tell yourself that your body can wait, that you first must make the kids their lunches. When it's time to watch your food portions, you'll again put your body on hold, supersizing your meal because you had a rough day.

But here's what happens when you fully accept and respect your body: You'll make your body your first priority *because* you love your kids, or spouse, or career. You'll make your body your first priority because you

know deep down that body acceptance and respect is the secret to better health, which is the secret to having more energy, love, and compassion for your family and your job. Putting your body first gives you the health and energy you need to become a better mother or father, spouse, friend, and employee.

I truly hope that you now realize the true magic that comes from fully accepting, respecting, and loving your body. This one distinction will lead you down a new path to success and health for a lifetime. Only when you take care of *you*, will you be able to give to those you love.

the respect test

So now that you're convinced that you must accept and respect your body right now rather than after you lose the weight, let's move on to the second myth that I mentioned in the beginning of this chapter: the false belief that you already accept and respect your body.

When I suggested to some of my clients that they first had to respect their bodies in order to succeed at weight loss, some of them told me that I was crazy. They said things like, "I already accept and respect my body."

I knew that simply wasn't the case because I had heard them

THE RESPECT TEST

Answer the following questions honestly. Then turn to page 26 to find out why answering "yes" means you don't fully respect and love your body.

1. Do you worry about what others think about your size?

2. Do you ever skip any meals, for any reason?

3. Do you want to lose weight only to improve your appearance rather than to improve your health?

4. Do you drink fewer than 8 glasses of water each day?

5. Do you have trouble finding time to exercise each day?

6. Do you feel you must lose weight in order to be sexy?

7. Do you think you must be smaller than a size 14 to be normal?

8. Do you try to avoid certain foods because you think they are bad and fattening?

9. Are you influenced by the media, friends, and family to be a smaller size?

10. Do you beat yourself up when you deviate from your healthy eating program?

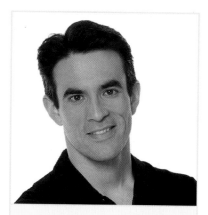

"If you don't fully accept and respect your current body, you will never treat it as the most precious gift that has ever been given to you."

curse their thighs or bellies many times before. I had heard their excuses about not exercising or eating healthfully, and I knew the excuses all boiled down to a lack of body acceptance and respect.

To help convince them that they needed to work on re-specting their bodies, I devel-oped a list of questions that I wanted them to answer honestly. The process helped my clients see that they didn't respect or ac-cept their bodies as much as they had thought.

I'd like you to take the same test that I developed for my clients. If you answer "yes" to any one of the questions on page 25, then you do not yet fully love and respect your body. Then, read on to find out why.

1. Do you worry about what others think about your size? Know that your body size does not determine your worthiness as a person. You earn love, re-spect, and admiration from others by your actions and per-sonality, not by the way you look. People who judge you by how you look are the ones who do not deserve *your* respect. Their judgment says more about their own internal dark-ness than it does about your ex-ternal body size.

2. Do you ever skip any meals, for any reason? Skip-ping meals is a form of body punishment. Many people skip meals to make up for excess calories that they ate the day be-fore or to try to lose weight quickly. But the tactic backfires. Meal skipping actually slows your metabolism, reducing the amount of calories you burn in a day. It also sends your blood sugar on a roller-coaster ride, setting you up for bingeing and overeating later on. (You'll learn more about this in chapter 6.) Be good to your body. Eat at least three sensible meals each day with healthy snacks in be-tween. Never punish your body with starvation.

3. Do you want to lose weight only to improve your appear-ance rather than to improve your health? Your outlook on life will dramatically improve the day you stop focusing on your outward appearance and instead learn to feel worthy from the inside out. Your health is what really matters. Getting fit and losing weight will help you to live longer, feel more energetic, sleep better, and get more out of life. You

critical secrets

Need a perfect example of a non-skinny woman with huge sex appeal? Take a look at Marilyn Monroe. Throughout her life she wore between a size 12 and 16, and she was one of the greatest sex symbols of modern times! If you don't believe me, rent a few of her films.

may also look better, too, but that shouldn't be your only goal.

4. Do you drink fewer than 8 glasses of water each day? When you truly respect your body, you will give it the fluids it needs to keep your energy levels high and your blood pumping smoothly. You'll learn more about the importance of water in chapter 6.

5. Do you have trouble finding time to exercise each day? Just as skipping meals is a form of body punishment, exercise is a form of body praise. You exercise to train your body to function at its highest potential. Everyone can find 8 minutes in a day to spend on his or her body. It takes body respect to turn a commitment to exercise into a reality.

6. Do you feel you must lose weight in order to be sexy? I've got news for you. The most tortured individuals are often the skinniest among us. Losing weight will not automatically make you feel sexy. Sex appeal comes from deep inside. Some of the skinniest men and women hate their bodies as much as some of the largest men and women—and feel just as unsexy as a result. When you build your inner confidence, you will feel and look sexy.

7. Do you think you must be smaller than a size 14 to be normal? Here's a statistic to help you see the light. About 65 million American women wear between a size 14 and 24. That's 1 out of every 2 to 3 women. The most common clothing size for women is 12 to 14. You are normal. Focus on getting more fit with the *8 Minutes in the Morning for Real Shapes, Real Sizes* program, and your body will naturally find its healthiest size and weight.

8. Do you try to avoid certain foods because you think they are bad and fattening? In order to lose weight, stop placing food into categories of "bad" and "good" and "fattening" and "slimming." Instead, focus on portion size. Of course, some foods are more heart-healthy than others, and you'll learn about those in chapter 6, but don't allow any food to make you feel bad about yourself. Once you release your guilt, you'll gain more control over your eating.

9. Are you influenced by the media, friends, and family to be a smaller size? For too many years, people have been hypnotized by outside influences to believe that women must be a size 6 to have a perfect body, or that men must

inside facts

It's hard to escape media images of superthin models and actresses. Know that ultrathin celebrities are the ones who do not lead normal lifestyles. According to some research, many of them are actually underweight—well below what's considered normal by the top health experts in our country. They subsist on superlow-calorie diets and exercise hours upon end to maintain their abnormally thin physiques. Promise yourself that you will aspire to lose only as much weight that is healthy and right for your body.

have ripped abs. This is not true. Some people are at their best and healthiest weight at size 12, 16, or 24.

10. Do you beat yourself up when you deviate from your healthy eating program? If you experience trouble sticking to an eating or exercise program, blame the program, not yourself. Weight loss is not a matter of willpower, but rather a matter of finding a program that works for your particular body size, needs, and lifestyle. It's not your fault, or your body's fault. It's the program's fault!

body respect 101

So how do you learn to accept, respect, and love your current body 100 percent, right now, extra weight and all? To learn how to do just that, I'd like you to try a very special two-step exercise that will quickly show you how to better accept, respect, and love your body and thus make weight loss a walk in the park!

step 1: get aware

Stop believing the old lies you have been consciously or subconsciously telling yourself about how your current body is not special enough, amazing enough, or precious enough to warrant your utmost attention and care *right now*. For example, if you are telling yourself, "Perhaps someday when it looks better (or younger or thinner), I will take better care of my body," you're telling yourself a lie.

I'd like you to uncover all of the damaging lies that you may be telling yourself, lies that will prevent you from fully accepting and respecting your body. To help you do that, I've listed 21 of the most common lies, ones that my clients have found limited their ability to succeed at any weight-loss plan.

1. "Losing weight is expensive." In reality, weight loss costs nothing. You don't need to buy expensive equipment or premade meals to lose weight. And think about this: The costs of not getting fit—heart disease, diabetes, arthritis—are much higher than the costs of starting a weight-loss program.

2. "I don't have enough time to exercise." You don't need a lot of time to get fit. You need only 8 minutes. That's right, just 8 minutes. Set your alarm 8 minutes earlier than usual and get up and just do it.

3. "I can overeat now and make up for these excess calories by eating less tomorrow." This is a form of procrastination, and it always results in disaster. Few people make up for the excess "tomorrow." And those who do eat less end up starving themselves and slowing their metabolisms. (You'll learn why this happens in chapter 6.) When you truly respect your body, you'll stick to healthful food portions all the time and never punish your body with starvation.

4. "I need to take care of others first. Once I meet their needs, then I can focus on myself." This is perhaps one of the most prevalent and most vicious lies out there. In reality, you can't take care of others until you have first taken care of yourself. When you neglect your mind and body, you eventually have nothing left to give. And if you suffer a heart attack from neglecting your body, eventually others will have to take care of you.

5. "Weight loss is not worth the effort. I'm just going to gain it all back anyway." I understand why you may feel this way, particularly if you have already lost and regained weight numerous times before. You must understand, however, that you're not to blame for those past failed attempts—the programs are at fault. To lose weight and keep it off, you must address the source of your problem. You must accept your body and heal your hungry heart. Once you do that, you will effortlessly lose the weight.

6. "My work is more important than my body." To quote a fairly well-known phrase: "No man ever said on his deathbed, 'I wish I had spent more time at the office.'" Yet, I would bet that plenty of people on their deathbeds had wished they had taken better care of their bodies.

7. "Weight doesn't matter. I am ugly at any size." Your body is an extraordinary machine that does extraordinary tasks every day. Once you learn to recognize that simple fact, you will realize that ugliness is a matter of perspective. If you focus on the amazing nature of your body—on your heart's ability to beat, on your muscles' ability to move, on your skin's ability to heal— then you will understand the inherent beauty of your body.

8. "Nobody loves me or cares about me, so why should I care about myself?" Perhaps one of the most perverse laws of human nature is that you must first love yourself before you can earn and receive love from others. Quite often, lack of self-love is what drives others from you. Think about it. Would you rather be around a depressed, sad, negative person or a confident, cheerful person? Once you become more confident, you'll find friends suddenly appearing in your life.

9. "I have already blown it today, so I might as well give up." You've never blown it until you've given up altogether. Just one overeating episode will not ruin your chance for success. For the same reason fat is so hard to lose, it is also hard to gain. It takes 3,500 *excess* calories in order to gain one pound of fat. That's a lot of food. Believe me, you've never eaten that much in one sitting!

THE GIFT THAT KEEPS ON GIVING

Not 100-percent convinced that your body is the most precious gift you have? Here are some facts about *your* amazing human body:

• Your heart beats 72 times a minute, more than 100,000 times a day, and roughly 2.5 billion times during your lifetime.

• Your heart weighs only 10 ounces, yet each day, it pumps 2,000 gallons of blood through 60,000 miles of blood vessels.

• Your kidneys completely filter all of your body's blood about 40 times each day.

• You breathe 14 times a minute and 7 million times a year without thinking about it.

• Your nose is capable of detecting 4,000 different odors.

• Each lung consists of more than 300 million microscopic sacs called alveoli where oxygen and carbon dioxide are exchanged in the blood. Spread out flat, a double layer of alveoli and capillaries from each lung would carpet a room 20 to 30 feet wide.

• Your stomach produces 2 to 3 pints of gastric juice every day. It takes more than 100 gallons of gastric juice to handle the food you eat in one year.

• Your eyes register 36,000 images an hour— and 864,000 a day.

• Muscles, if they could work together and pull in one direction, equal 25 tons of pulling power.

• All of these processes are done in a body that's made up of about 80 percent water.

10. "I work hard. I deserve to eat as much as I want." If you work hard, you deserve to pamper yourself, that's true. But overeating is a form of body punishment, not a form of pampering. I suggest you treat yourself to a

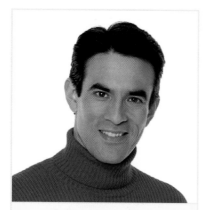

"I know from my most successful 8-minute marvels that real weight loss only happens once your body becomes your highest priority."

massage, a warm bath, or a long talk with an old friend instead of treating yourself to food.

11. "I am fine on the inside. That's all that matters." Both the inside and the outside of your body matter. Excess weight—on the outside—weakens and sickens the inside of your body. Take care of the outside of your body by losing weight, and the inside—your heart, lungs, and blood vessels—will become healthier and stronger.

12. "One day of not caring is not going to matter." The problem with this thinking is that 1 day turns into 2 days which turns into 3 days, then 4, and so on. Start caring about your body *today*.

13. "My husband/wife loves me no matter what my size." I'm sure your spouse loves you, but this isn't about your spouse. This is about you. You should lose weight to make your life better, to improve your body, to feel more energetic and healthy, and to make your life easier. Of course, those around you will benefit, but you are the one that counts the most.

14. "Food is the only friend that can lift my spirits or remove the ache of loneliness." Plenty of things—besides food—can help you heal your hungry

heart. You'll learn about them in chapter 3.

15. "I don't want to offend my friends by not indulging with them." My mother used to say, "If your friend jumped off a bridge, would you do it too?" Overeating hurts you just as much as using recreational drugs. If your friends are offended that you want to take better care of your body, they are not really your friends.

16. "I'm old. All old people are fat." It's true that many people gain weight as they age as a result of a slower metabolism. If you strength train, however, you can keep your metabolism from slowing down in the first place. You'll learn more about this in chapter 4.

17. "I'm still young. I can lose the weight later." The statistics are stacked against you on this one. Most people tend to *gain* weight as they get older, not lose it. The best time to lose weight is right now!

18. "I can eat as much as my 6-foot-2-inch husband." You probably know that this isn't true—as much as you want it to be so. Many women tell me that they gained weight when they were first married and began eating the same food portions as their husbands. Your husband has more muscle mass and is probably

MY TOP 3 LIMITING BELIEFS

Write down the top three lies or limiting beliefs you've told yourself in the past that resulted in you not treating your body with the attention and respect it deserves.

My #1 lie: _____

The negative consequences of believing this lie:

_____

_____

_____

_____

My #2 lie: _____

The negative consequences of believing this lie:

_____

_____

_____

_____

My #3 lie: _____

The negative consequences of believing this lie:

_____

_____

_____

_____

taller, and he therefore burns more calories each day than you do. You must stick to smaller food portions in order to lose weight.

19. "My metabolism is terrible." This may be true. After many years of dieting, your metabolism may be much slower than it used to be. You can rev it up, however, with strength training. You'll learn more about this in chapter 4.

20. "I'm genetically meant to be overweight." This is only a half-truth. Some people do carry what scientists call a "thrifty gene," which makes their bodies resist burning fat. It only means,

however, that you'll have to work a little harder than someone without this gene in order to lose weight and keep it off.

21. "I'm too fat to exercise." This lie is what led me to develop this book. Certain types of exercise may not be best suited for your body. But I know that you'll be able to comfortably perform the exercises in my program. I tested them on full-figured women. They work.

Did any of those lies resonate with you? Have you found yourself using them to make excuses for not exercising or eating healthful food portions? Do you

have even more lies buried deep inside? Take a moment right now to think about what you've told yourself in the past that led to overeating or not exercising. Were you lying to yourself?

To get fully aware of your damaging, negative, and false beliefs, I want you write down *your* top three limiting beliefs on page 31 that you have consciously or subconsciously told yourself, lies that resulted in your not believing that your body was special enough, amazing enough, or precious enough to warrant your highest attention and care. Feel free to borrow a few from those I mentioned earlier.

ULTIMATE REFERENCES

Use these ultimate references or others like them to remind yourself to put your body first.

- I have only one body. I cannot get another one if I ruin this one.
- My body is the only real instrument to live my life's purpose.
- My body is my life. When it is gone, so am I.
- I am smart, and I realize the power of this belief.
- My body is my vehicle to being an active parent.
- My body is the most important instrument I have to contribute to our world.
- My nose allows me to enjoy the amazing aromas of a beautiful rose.

- My nervous system allows me to bliss out with a foot massage.
- My eyes allow me to see the beautiful smile on my baby's face.
- My amazing ears allow me to hear the relaxing sound of the ocean's waves.
- My body runs almost automatically and can heal itself.
- My arms allow me to hug and show my love for my friends, family, and kids.
- My legs allow me to dance, play, and travel this world.
- My body is God's temple.

renee hinton lost 44 pounds

I had high blood pressure and was taking medicine for it. I had high cholesterol, sleep apnea, and bad knees. I knew that I had to do something soon, but what? I never before had been able to stick to a diet for any length of time since gaining weight after age 60. Jorge helped me lose 44 pounds!

"I no longer have knee pain."

I can walk like I did during my 30s (and I just celebrated my 70th birthday!). I am now able to wear so many nice clothes and do so many more things.

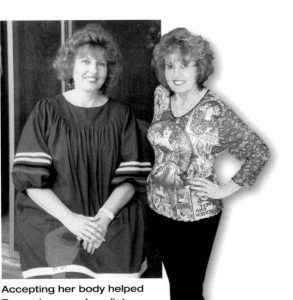

Accepting her body helped Renee improve her diet.

After you write down your top three limiting beliefs, write down the consequence of believing these old dis-empowering beliefs. And know that dissatisfaction can be a powerful spark that gets you to take action and change your behaviors forever.

Once you've completed the limiting-beliefs exercise, you're ready to take another step on your journey to body respect. To fully acknowledge that your three negative beliefs are no longer a part of you, I want you to do something symbolic. Take a thick, black marker and ink out those three old beliefs with your pen. Yes, draw on top of them. Cover them up. Put a big xxx over them. This may seem like a simple, and maybe even silly, exercise, but believe me, it will symbolically help you to delete those same lies from your brain's hard drive.

By doing this, you will be signaling to your brain and subconscious that you are no longer willing to be ruled by these lies. As the words disappear, so will those damaging beliefs! You will feel empowered and invigorated. You will be free. Don't continue to read this book until you have done this exercise. This physical act of destroying those old beliefs will impact your future success for the better. You will almost feel reborn.

step 2: replace the junk with a gem

Now that you have cleared out your emotional closet of the junk, it is now time to replace that junk with a true gem: empowering beliefs that will change your life and how you treat your body forever. Ready? Simply replace those three old limiting beliefs with the following power pledge:

"My current body is the most precious gift I have ever been given."

To fully commit that pledge to memory, write down the positive consequences of believing this

MY POWER PLEDGE POSTER

My current body is the most precious gift I have ever been given.
I am very grateful for it and will accept it, respect it, and love it 100 percent each day.

The positive consequences of believing this:

_____

_____

_____

_____

_____

_____

_____

My 10 ultimate references (Why this pledge is true. See page 32 for ideas.):

1. _____

2. _____

3. _____

4. _____

5. _____

6. _____

7. _____

8. _____

9. _____

10. _____

gem on the Power Pledge Poster, opposite. For example, you might write:

• "I will treat my body as a top priority."

• "I will make sure to exercise my body on a regular basis."

• "I will feed my body properly."

• "I will finally lose the extra weight."

To strengthen your pledge, I want you to support it with 10

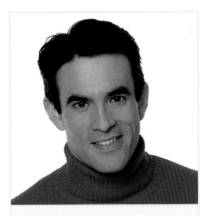

"Promise yourself that you will aspire to lose only as much weight that is healthy and right for your body."

ultimate references. These are 10 ideas that make the power pledge completely real for you.

To create your ultimate references, ask yourself this simple question: "Why is this true?" In other words, "Why is my current body truly the most precious gift I have ever been given?" Write your answers on your Power Pledge Poster in the spaces provided.

To help get you started, refer to page 32 for some great ultimate references that some of my clients have used.

Now that you've listed your 10 ultimate references, I want you to finish creating your Power Pledge Poster. Please turn to it again, right now, and fill in the rest of the blanks.

Once you complete your Power Pledge Poster, photocopy it three times, and place the posters in three spots in your house. I highly recommend posting it on your nightstand and in the bathroom, so you can see it when you first get up, and in the kitchen, so you can see it whenever you feel tempted to overeat or skip your Cruise Moves.

Your poster will serve as a powerful reminder to put your body first. One of my clients, Renee Hinton, who is very proud that she is "70 years young," makes sure to look at

your questions

Why can't I wait until I lose the weight to accept my body?

Well, it just doesn't work that way. Feedback from my millions of online clients proves that you first must accept your body and then lose the weight. It simply doesn't work in the reverse. Once you accept your body, you will treat it like a gift and prioritize your body's needs. Only then will you be able to lose weight and keep it off!

her poster every morning. She reads her ultimate references, such as "My body is the only body I will ever have" and "My body is the vehicle that lets me walk, talk, think, learn, breathe, love, and live life to the fullest." When she looks at her poster, she's reminded that her body allows her to do all the things she loves, such as going to the theater and visiting her family and friends.

Doing this every morning helps her not only to do her 8-minute Cruise Moves but also to follow her Cruise Down Plate. "I used to eat too much fast food and too many sweets. I didn't consume enough vitamins and

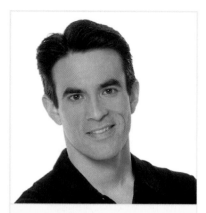

"Focus on getting more fit with this program, and your body will naturally find its healthiest size and weight."

minerals, and, as a result, suffered from high blood pressure and high cholesterol," she said. "But once I unconditionally accepted my body, I instantly started watching what I ate." (You can read the rest of her amazing story on page 33.)

Before we move on to the next chapter, remember that it is essential for you to realize that the first secret to real weight loss is to unconditionally accept and thus respect your body 100 percent, right now, no matter what your current size. If you don't fully respect your current body, I can assure you that you will never truly treat it as the most precious gift that has ever been given to you.

So my specific challenge to you right now is that you photocopy your Power Pledge Poster and put it in three places. Review it each morning and each night before bed for a minimum of 28 days!

By doing this, your health will consistently become your number one priority. You will effortlessly make the best decisions for your body, and you will discover the most important secret to finally shedding the pounds and keeping them off forever.

3

The Second Secret to Weight-Loss Success

Heal Your Hungry Heart and Eliminate Emotional Eating

the people solution

Now that you've mastered the first secret to successful weight loss—accepting your body no matter what your size—you're ready to tackle the second step on your *8 Minutes in the Morning for Real Shapes, Real Sizes* journey. You're ready to heal your hungry heart. What do I mean specifically?

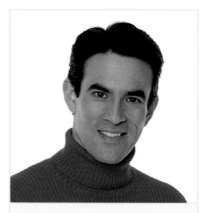

To be successful at losing weight, you must discover how to stop using food as your preferred emotional supporter and instead replace it with a more attractive alternative—one that has no negative side effects on your waistline. My goal for you in this chapter is simple. I'm going to teach you a smarter, more effi-cient, and calorie-free method that will help you to experience the ultimate sense of support and comfort without any food at all. It's a revolutionary answer for emotional eating that I call The People Solution.

By enacting The People Solution, you will instantly feel unwavering strength. Your life will feel more fulfilled and whole, without the need for food as comfort. And most important, you will eliminate emotional eating, thus removing the number one roadblock to your weight-loss success!

> "The true source of your weight challenge stems from a hurtful void or emptiness in your life."

your "8 minute" edge

By activating The People Solution, you will:

• Instantly feel more nurtured and supported

• Make your daily quality of life feel richer, deeper, and more fulfilling without the need for food

• Eliminate emotional eating, thus removing the number one roadblock to your weight-loss success!

why you overeat

Emotional eating is only a symptom. The true source of your weight challenge stems from a hurtful void or emptiness in your life. It stems from your hungry heart.

In the past, when you overate when you where not hungry, food helped fill a void and numb a pain. Food made you feel supported and comforted.

I often ask my new clients, "What makes you feel this void or emptiness?" I ask them to close their eyes and carefully think back to when they first started to put on weight, to think about what had changed in their lives.

For one of my clients, Jennifer, that change came in the form of stress. She was the primary breadwinner of the home. She worked full-time at a demanding job and then came home to take care of her husband and children.

Her husband not only didn't work but he also didn't bother to clean or cook or help out in any way. Food became her only escape. She told me that when she ate, she *felt* better. Yet, once she enacted The People Solution, she found something better than food to support her, and she lost 35 pounds as a result!

Another client, Susan, lost 2½ pounds during her first week with me just by implementing The People Solution. Susan and

I had met for the first time a few weeks earlier, when I had asked her that crucial question: "When do you first remember gaining weight?"

"At age 25, when I went back to school," she said. "I was unhappily married to a controlling, abusive husband who didn't want me to go to school. Due to financial problems, I had to work full-time along with taking a full load of classes. Plus, my husband offered no help at home, so

BREAK THE EMOTIONAL EATING CYCLE

As the chart below displays, The People Solution will help you to break the emotional eating cycle once and for all.

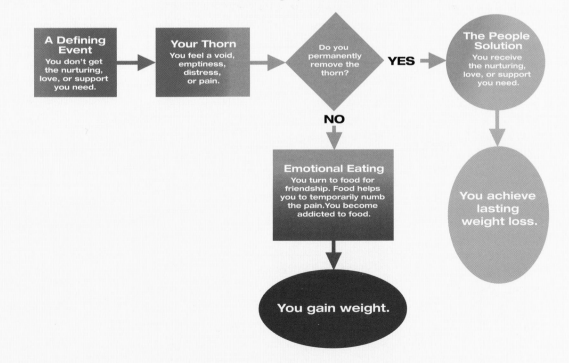

something had to go. That something was close ties to my friends." As Susan became more and more isolated, the pounds crept on.

Susan and I talked for a while about the importance of friendship and support. She promised to start e-mailing a few women she met at JorgeCruise.com, particularly whenever she felt the urge to eat to soothe her emotions. And that's when the pounds started coming off.

Many of my clients have told me of similar experiences, of a particular event in their lives that made them feel hurt, alone, or sad. Without people to turn to for comfort, they began turning to food to soothe the pain. Yet, once they brought nurturing friendships and support back into their lives, they were able to eliminate their dependence on

inside facts

The best solution is people.

If you read my first book, *8 Minutes in the Morning*, you know that I shared my basic system for eliminating emotional eating. The People Solution is the next phase, my most powerful solution, to eliminating emotional eating.

food and finally lose the weight and keep it off.

My sister, Marta, linked her problems to grade school. In a well-intentioned attempt to improve my sister's education, my mother transferred Marta from one school to another. As soon as Marta established a set of friends at one school, Mom pulled her out and enrolled her in another. She attended five different schools in 5 years!

As a result, Marta rarely had close childhood friends. She turned to food to soothe her loneliness. As I explained in chapter 1, she lost weight only after she developed a strong network of friends.

Another example is my good friend Emme, who told me that she first began gaining weight at age 10. Her stepfather was obsessed with his weight of more than 300 pounds. To keep Emme from following in his footsteps, he began weighing her and her mom once a week and writing the results on a chart on the wall. He also told her to strip down to her underwear and then drew circles around her thighs, hips, and arms to point out her trouble spots.

She felt ashamed. As a result, she did just what her stepfather was trying to prevent. She turned to food to nurture herself and suppress her emotions.

Then there's Erin McLeod, whom you met in chapter 1. When I asked her to think back to her first problems with weight, she thought back to age 7, when her parents divorced. Both parents spent their evenings partying and socializing. Then at age 30, Erin was married and became pregnant. She had one baby and then another. Her husband went out every night, leaving her alone with the kids.

"My only companion was food," she told me. "I finally realized that what I felt when my husband left me alone was the same thing I felt when my parents left me alone. I felt lonely, unloved, and unwanted."

Once Erin enacted The People Solution, she broke the cycle. She left her husband, went back to school, and lost 75 pounds. "I deserve to be loved and respected," she later said. "I will never again allow myself to be taken for granted or made to feel unloved or unwanted."

thorns in your heart

The examples go on and on. Some of my clients remember being sexually abused and then turning to food not only to numb the pain but also to hide their bodies. Others turned to food out of boredom or fear or sadness. I often refer to such painful and distressful events as thorns.

Some thorns, such as a rape or physical abuse, are big and hurt very deeply. Others, such as loneliness or boredom, may seem smaller, but they still leave their mark. You might have just one thorn or you might have many, but if you eat emotionally, your heart was pierced by a thorn at some point in your life.

You see, we humans are hard-wired to avoid pain and seek out pleasure. Any psychologist will tell you that. So to avoid the pain of these thorns and continue to seek out pleasure, where did you turn? What became your number one way to numb the pain? What became your best friend? What became your number one comforter and emotional supporter?

Food is likely the answer to all of those questions.

Yet food is only a temporary pain-numbing solution. Think of it as a cream that you would dab on your hand to remove the pain of a wound. Eventually the cream wears off, and the pain returns. To keep the pain under control, you must apply more and more cream.

And here is the most critical thing you must understand. This is where your life is about to change forever. You must clearly

see that you can no longer use food as a temporary pain remover. No weight-loss program will ever work if you are addicted to food as comfort. You must first make a shift deep inside, a shift that will help you zero in on the source of your problem, a shift that will help you to stop relying on food for comfort. That shift will happen when you activate The People Solution.

how the people solution works

You will find The People Solution a thousand times more attractive than food. The People Solution will give you the comfort, nurturing, and support you need to break your addiction to food.

Think about it. In the past, when you ate and you were not hungry, what were you feeling? Perhaps boredom, stress, loneliness, sadness, anger, frustration, inadequacy, or hopelessness? No matter what you were feeling, instead of turning to food for comfort, if you could have turned to someone to support and nurture you, you would not have turned to food.

We all need nurturing to make us feel strong and supported. Nurturing in the form of someone saying, "I can see you

critical secrets

The People Solution includes three simple steps:

step 1: Become your own greatest friend
step 2: Get your inner team to support you
step 3: Expand your buddy team

are not feeling well. Tell me about your day. How are you feeling?" Nurturing in the form of a shoulder to cry on, a hug, or someone who is really interested in what you are saying. Nurturing in the form of a friend to take a walk with or a soft whisper in your ear saying, "I understand what you're going through." Or nurturing in the form of a parent or spouse saying, "I love you and approve of you the way you are, no matter what."

Unfortunately, few of us get this kind of nurturing throughout our lives. I can guess that at some point, someone was not there to help you and give you the nurturing you needed. Perhaps your mom or dad was too busy working, your spouse was too tired to listen and spend time with you, or your best friend moved away. Yet, the need for this kind of nurturing is extremely powerful. It's one of the most powerful human needs, and we all have them.

You see, the human heart absolutely needs nurturing and support. Probably the most compelling demonstration of this phenomenon comes from research done with babies. As babies, if we don't receive enough nurturing, comfort, and support from a parent or other caregiver, the result is a chemical deficiency and immune system inefficiency that can lead to severe handicap or even death. Doctors call it "failure to thrive" syndrome.

The hunger for this kind of nurturing and comfort is so strong that if we don't find it in people, we search for it in other forms. This search can lead some people to drugs. For others, the search might lead to alcohol. And for you, your search likely led you to *food*.

Until now, you've spent most of your life healing your pain with a food solution, instead of The People Solution. You might have found a best friend in a dish, in a bowl, on a plate, or in a bag of chips because food never let you down. Food gave you a kind of unconditional and unwavering support.

So what's the alternative source we should use to fill our emotional voids with the nurturing we need? Well, as I said earlier, it's *people*! Yes, people.

People are your most powerful resource. The feeling of needing to fill yourself up with food will instantly disappear once you fill your hungry heart with nurturing, comfort, and support from people.

So now it's your turn to join Jennifer, Susan, Marta, Emme, Erin, and countless others. It's your turn to activate The People Solution and walk away from emotional eating once and for all. Let's get started!

step 1

The first person in The People Solution must be you. Yes, you must first become your greatest friend and ally. Why? I'll answer that in a moment.

become your own greatest friend

First let me ask you a few questions.

- Who feeds you?
- Who determines whether you exercise in the morning?
- Who puts you to sleep?
- Who controls your life?

The answers to those questions is you. Yes, you. You control your life. You make the decision to exercise and eat right. You decide when to go to sleep and when to wake. You're in control.

I'll say it again: You must become your greatest ally and friend. Only then will you ignite your deepest motivation to take better care of yourself. Only then will you treat yourself with the greatest care and respect. Only then will others feel more able to unconditionally nurture, comfort, and support you.

To become your own greatest friend, you must do three things.

- Accept your current self (no matter what)
- Ignite your deepest motivation
- Use a journal to express your feelings

accept your current self

You're already ahead of the game on this one because we covered this in chapter 2. In that chapter,

elizabeth callaway lost 30 pounds

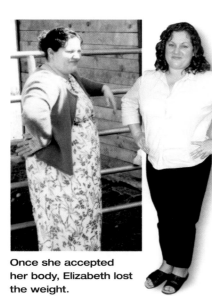

Once she accepted her body, Elizabeth lost the weight.

I have a hectic schedule with two children ages 3 and 6, and my son just started preschool. It is challenging to get everybody dressed, fed, groomed, and off to school. I work between 9 A.M. and 2 P.M., but I've still managed to lose 30 pounds with Jorge's plan. I make time each morning for my Cruise Moves and an extra minute or two of stretching afterwards. I always do it while I am still in my pajamas, so nothing gets in the way.

"Doing the exercises gives me a boost of energy."

I want to be strong and healthy. I want to be active and a good role model for my children. I am taking back my life, and being fit and confident is a vital part of it.

you learned the first secret to successful weight loss—to unconditionally accept and respect your body 100 percent right now (no matter what your size).

Once you fully accept and respect your body, you will begin to treat it as the greatest gift you've ever received. Only then will you find the effortless motivation to follow my Cruise Down Plate and Cruise Moves routines. You can't enact The People Solution until you have completed this important step. So before you move on, make sure you have completed your Power Pledge Poster and all of the exercises in chapter 2. This is critical to your success.

I think Elizabeth Callaway, one of my clients, best summed up this important concept. "I have always pushed myself to be something different than I was," she told me. "Even when I was a size 6, I wanted to be a size 4. Now I wish I would have appreciated myself and treated myself better. Once I decided to unconditionally accept, love, and appreciate myself, I began making better choices, making time for myself, and asking my family for help. I feel so much happier and better about myself." (Read more about Elizabeth above.)

As Elizabeth's story clearly shows, acceptance is the first step toward healing your hungry

heart. You must take each step to successful weight loss in the right order to see lasting results.

ignite your deepest motivation

Once you learn to accept your current body, you are ready to ignite your deepest motivation. Doing so starts by establishing a specific goal.

My good friend and mentor, Anthony Robbins, taught me years ago that we can never easily achieve success without a target or goal. Let's say you wanted your best friend to attend a very special event for you, such as a dinner party at a fancy restaurant. What kind of a friend would you be if you purposely did not give your friend the street address? Not a very good one because, without the address, your friend would never arrive.

It's the same with you. You must now be a good friend to yourself and give yourself the street address of success. You must give yourself a very specific goal for your weight loss. This goal will help to ignite your motivation to lose weight, eat right, and do your Cruise Moves each morning.

As Robyn McAteer, one of my clients, put it, "Knowing my goal weight and goal date keeps me motivated. It gives me a clear visual of what I am working towards. In the past, I used to set a high goal. But now that I have learned to accept and love my body, I've changed that goal to one that's more realistic and attainable. That, of course, means my date has gotten closer, as well." (Read more about Robyn below.)

Elizabeth, the successful client whom I mentioned earlier, set her goal date as her son's fourth birthday. "I had never before actually sat down and figured out how long it would take me to lose the weight I wanted to lose," she said. "It is amazing to break it down and have it become a reality."

So here is what you must do. Turn to "My Healthy Weight," opposite, and determine your healthy weight. This will not only help you to pinpoint a goal weight and goal date but also help you to set minigoals along the way, which will give you short-term targets to focus on.

If you have a lot of weight to lose, your overall goal date may seem very far away. Losing weight at a safe 2 pounds a week means that it will take you 15 weeks to lose 30 pounds, 50 weeks to lose 100 pounds, and 100 weeks to lose 200 pounds. I know that 15, 50, and 100 weeks seem like a very long time. That's why I want you to set shorter goals along the way. These minigoals will give you reasons to celebrate your success.

(continued on page 49)

robyn mcateer lost 66 pounds

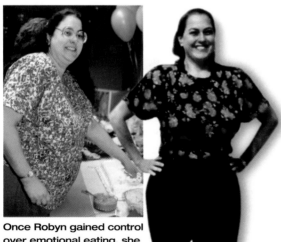

Once Robyn gained control over emotional eating, she lost weight.

Thanks to The People Solution, I have lost something much more important than 66 pounds. I have lost feelings of regret, unworthiness, hopelessness, and loneliness.

"I feel such a sense of freedom now that food no longer controls me."

Food no longer controls my thoughts. I will never regain this weight. I will no longer live in the past, but rather, I will look forward to my future with hope and determination. I am an ordinary person determined to have extraordinary success.

MY HEALTHY WEIGHT

To find your healthy weight, find your age and height on the chart below. You know yourself better than anyone else does, so select a number that is realistic for you. Subtract that number from your current weight. That's your weight-loss goal.

My weight-loss goal: _____

Now let's figure out a target date for achieving this goal. If you stick with me as your coach, you will lose about 2 pounds per week, which is what doctors recommend. If you have 70 or more pounds to lose, you might lose more than 2 pounds each week for the first month. Regardless, take the number you wrote on the line above and divide it by 2. This number equals the number of weeks it will take you to reach your goal weight. Consult a calendar and find the exact date you will achieve your goal weight.

Date I will reach my ideal weight: _____

Now, I want you to set three minigoals. Divide the number of weeks it will take you to achieve your goal weight by 4. For example, if you have 50 pounds to lose, it will take you 25 weeks to reach your goal. Divide 25 by 4, and you'll get 6. That's how many weeks you'll space your minigoals apart. Consult a calendar and write the dates of your minigoals in the spaces below.

My minigoals:

1. _____

2. _____

3. _____

I hereby promise to review this page every morning to keep me motivated and supported.

Signature: _____

your weight chart

Height (ft/in.)	Weight (lb)		Height (ft/in.)	Weight (lb)	
	19–34 yr	35+ yr		19–34 yr	35+ yr
5'0"	97–128	108–38	5'8"	125–64	138–78
5'1"	101–32	111–43	5'9"	129–69	142–83
5'2"	104–37	115–48	5'10"	132–74	146–88
5'3"	107–41	119–52	5'11"	136–79	151–94
5'4"	111–46	122–57	6'0"	140–84	155–99
5'5"	114–50	126–62	6'1"	144–89	159–205
5'6"	118–55	130–67	6'2"	148–95	164–210
5'7"	121–60	134–72	6'3"	152–200	168–216

SOURCE: U.S. Department of Health and Human Services, Dietary Guidelines for Americans

MY "BEFORE" AND "AFTER" PHOTOS

Your "before" and "after" photos will help motivate you to stay focused on your weight-loss goal.
Review both of these pages each day to *prevent* emotional eating.
Take your "before" photos right now and paste them on this page.

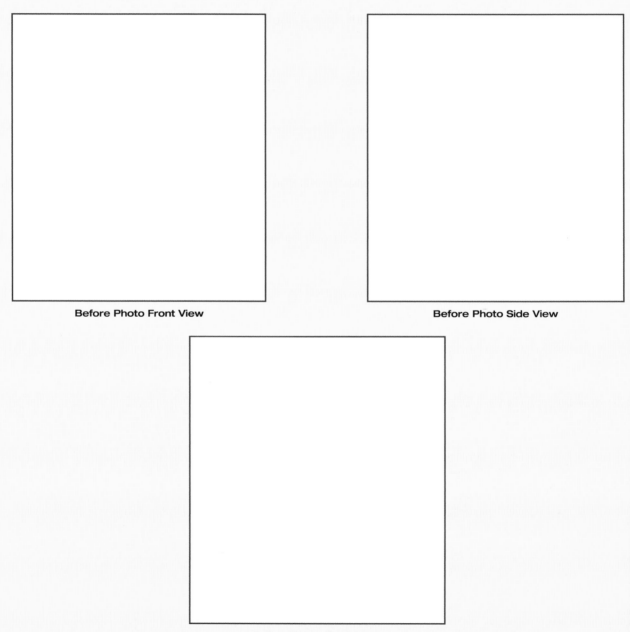

Before Photo Front View

Before Photo Side View

Before Photo Back View

Don't wait to see your future body! Go to www.jorgecruise.com/futurebody
and print out your "after" photos right now.

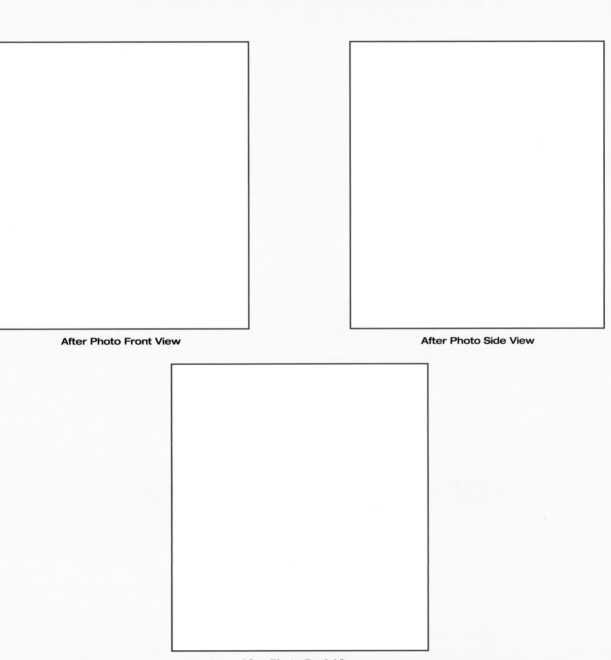

After Photo Front View

After Photo Side View

After Photo Back View

A DAY IN THE LIFE
OF THE FUTURE ME

In the space provided, describe a typical day at your goal weight, including details about your appearance, energy, and overall lifestyle. You can handwrite your essay here in this book, or, if you prefer, type it up on your computer and print it out and paste it in the space provided.

Review this page daily to prevent emotional eating. Keep it by your nightstand and read it when you wake in the morning. Or, take a tip from one of my clients and read your essay into a tape recorder. Then listen to the audiocassette as you do your Cruise Moves or while driving in your car.

_____

_____

_____

_____

_____

_____

_____

_____

_____

_____

_____

_____

_____

_____

_____

_____

A DAY IN THE LIFE
OF THE FUTURE JACQUI

"I feel the sun peeking through my bedroom window, and I'm ready to spring out of bed 30 minutes before the alarm rings, full of energy and life. I walk down my lush tropical garden path to the beach and take a brisk stroll as the sun rises. I then sit down in the sand to relish my quiet time. The sand is still warm from yesterday's sun. The early seagulls are diving for their breakfast. . . .

"I run up the stairs of my beachfront, multilevel home and effortlessly complete my Cruise Moves. It's become so natural, that it's just like breathing now. After my 8-minute recharge, I start my day of freedom. After fueling my strong body with healthy breakfast foods, I hop into the shower and get my face ready for my makeup. I don't have to apply as much makeup as I used to. As I wash my face, I notice how my face has changed. My Native American high cheek-bones are very pronounced. My almond brown eyes sparkle and are the focal point of my face. My mouth is more proportionate with my face now. My lips look fuller and my smile looks brighter, framed by my small oval face that no longer dons the double chin. . . .

"I slip into my little black dress that accents my svelte curves. I don't wear a jacket. It's a business look yet a bit on the flirty side, complimented by high-heeled pumps.

"I get into my new convertible retro Thunderbird, and I'm off to the studio to produce my syndicated children's show. . . . " (See her "before" and "after" photos on page 77.)

And you should celebrate! For your long-term goal and for each short-term goal, I want you to reward yourself. But pick a reward that has nothing to do with food. Maybe you'll treat yourself with a manicure or pedicure, a massage, a day at a spa, a shopping spree, or a trip. Pick a reward that will motivate you to stay on track.

See your future self. Now you'll continue to ignite your deepest motivation by creating a clear visual picture of your future body at your goal weight.

First, take three "before" photos of yourself, one for front, side, and back views of your body, in your regular clothes (unless you want to be in a bathing suit). After you take those three photos, paste them on page 46.

Your before photos will serve as constant reminders of how much progress you've made. During a weight-loss journey, it's easy to feel discouraged, to feel as if you haven't really lost much weight. Whenever you feel that way, just take a look at your before photos. They don't lie!

Now for the exciting part—your "after" photos. You don't actually have to lose the weight to see your future body. Just go to www.jorgecruise.com/futurebody. This incredible online tool will help you create a photo of yourself at your future ideal weight! It is a revolutionary virtual photo technology created by a company in Canada called MyVirtualModel.

Simply follow the directions online, and soon you'll see the future you. Then print out three photos of your front, side, and back. Once you print these out, paste them in the after spots on page 47. I hope you find these photos as exciting as my clients have!

(Note: If you don't have online access, you can use photos of you from before you gained the extra weight, or you can choose photos from magazines of realistic women such as Emme who are at your goal weight. Paste these photos on page 47.)

These photos will serve as a powerful motivating force. Along with the Power Pledge Poster you created in chapter 2, review your before-and-after photos each morning before you start your day. They will help keep you motivated and focused.

Once you paste your after photos into this book, you're ready to move on to the final task in igniting your deepest motivation.

Describe the future you. Now that you can see the future you, you're ready to describe the future you. On page 48, I want you to describe the ideal day in the life of the future you. Starting from the moment you get out of bed to the moment you go to sleep, describe a typical day in your life *after you've reached your goal weight*. Describe comments people say to you, the new people in your life, the clothes you're wearing, and, most important, your feelings of joy and happiness. Describe your

new body in every detail, from your head to your toes.

You may at first think that this exercise seems silly, but trust me. It will serve as a powerful motivator. You get what you focus on. Too often, people concentrate on their current weight, constantly focusing on the reasons why they are overweight. But this doesn't get you anywhere.

If you focus on you at your *healthy weight*, then you will point yourself in the right direction toward achieving your goal. As motivational guru Stephen Covey has said, you must begin with the end in mind. All successful endeavors, he says, are created twice. You must first create a mental picture of what you want *before* you can create a physical picture. In other words, if you *see* your body and your life at your goal weight, you will achieve your goal weight.

That's why describing a day in your future life is so powerful. It helps you to clearly see the future you.

But don't just take my word for it. This exercise has worked for many of my most successful clients. For example, Jacqui Poor reviews her Day in the Life of the Future Me essay *every day*. She told me that the essay helps to paint a powerful picture that keeps her motivated.

Jacqui's essay is too long for me to print in its entirety, but you can find an excerpt on page 49 to give you an idea of what to write. Once you complete your own Day in the Life of the Future Me essay, you may move on to the final step in igniting your deepest motivation.

use a journal to express your feelings

Finally, you're ready to learn about your final secret to becoming your own greatest friend. This secret lies in putting pen to paper.

Before you do anything else, I want you to find a notebook that you can use as your weight-loss journal. Write in this notebook *every day*, describing everything from your feelings to your weight-loss successes and challenges. I want this journal to go with you wherever you go.

Keeping a journal is without a doubt one of the most powerful tools you can use to express your feelings. Writing down your thoughts and feelings can be incredibly therapeutic. For example, research shows that those who write down their feelings tend to improve *both* their emotional and physical health. In one study, people with arthritis who wrote about their feelings experienced less joint pain!

It's as if something magical happens when you put pen to paper. The process of writing down your thoughts acts like a powerful salve to heal your mind, body, and soul. It's almost as if someone is right there listening to you and offering support.

Turn to your notebook, along with your buddies (more on that later), whenever you feel the urge to eat. Turn to it whenever you feel stressed, angry, sad, tense, depressed, guilty, or lonely. Let your journal serve as a friend, lending a shoulder for you to cry on whenever you need one, serving as a substitute for food.

I believe so much in the power of journaling that I've included space for you to write down your thoughts, feelings, successes, and challenges on each day of your 28-day challenge in chapter 7. *Feel free to write in this book.* That's what it's here for. Let it serve as that extra support you need to express yourself, emptying the deepest negative emotions out of your body and putting them onto paper.

step 2

Now that you've completed the exercises needed to help you become your own greatest friend, you are ready to move on to Step 2 of The People Solution.

get your inner team to support you

For this important step, you will need to establish a weight-loss support network—your inner team. Your inner team can include family, coworkers, church members, and, of course, your good friends. You should choose people that allow you to feel comfortable communicating your feelings. These people must be nonjudgmental.

Think of seven people whom you'd like to invite to become members of your support team. List them in the space provided on page 52. For now, leave Kind and Contact Info blank. (If you don't have seven people you feel comfortable asking, then fill in as many as you can.) Your buddies must truly care about you and be willing to listen to and support you.

Now, here's how each of the categories in the Kind column work.

E-mail buddies. You will e-mail these buddies anytime you feel you are about to eat to soothe your emotions. In your e-mails, share that you almost turned to food to soothe your emotions. Tell them what you are feeling and why.

For example, you might write: "I feel very overwhelmed and depressed. My boss just gave me too much work to finish by 5 P.M. today, and my husband never helps me with the kids when I come home. I feel like crap, and I want to grab a candy bar."

Ask your buddies to respond within 24 hours with a support e-mail. This e-mail should comfort you, which is why it's so important to choose nonjudgmental buddies. Return to your support team list on page 52 and write "e-mail buddy" in the Kind column next to three of the seven members of your support team. Then under the Contact Info column, write their e-mail addresses.

Phone buddies. You will call your phone buddies anytime you feel you are about to eat to

MY SUPPORT TEAM

List the seven people on your support team in the spaces provided.

Name	**Kind**	**Contact Info**
1. _____	_____	_____
2. _____	_____	_____
3. _____	_____	_____
4. _____	_____	_____
5. _____	_____	_____
6. _____	_____	_____
7. _____	_____	_____

Next you will place those seven people into the following buddy groups:

- 3 e-mail buddies
- 3 phone buddies
- 1 accountability buddy

Don't forget to give all the buddies on your inner team a copy of your Power Pledge Poster, your healthy weight page, and your Day in the Life of the Future Me essay. These tools will help familiarize your buddies with your goal and your commitment.

soothe your emotions. Your phone buddies will serve as a lifeline. Whenever you need immediate support, you will call the first buddy on the list. If that buddy isn't home, you'll try the next, and so on.

Go back to your support team list above, and write "phone buddy" in the Kind column next to three of the seven people listed. Then, in the column under Contact Info, write their home, work, and cell phone numbers.

An accountability buddy. Your accountability buddy needs to keep you accountable for your goal, each week, no matter what. Also, this buddy must already be living the lifestyle you want. This means that your accountability buddy must be healthy and fit, someone who serves as a role model to you.

Your accountability buddy must be available to talk with you for 30 minutes once a week, preferably on Sunday nights or Monday mornings. During these talks, re-

SAMPLE BUDDY LETTERS

Try this letter when you contact your e-mail buddies.

Hi Chris,

I consider you one of my good friends, and I need your help and support. I am committed to losing weight so that I can improve my health. I am using Jorge Cruise's *8 Minutes in the Morning for Real Shapes, Real Sizes* weight-loss program. To be successful at losing the weight, I need three "e-mail buddies." I would be honored if you would serve as one of these buddies.

If you agree to serve as my e-mail buddy, your job would be to check your e-mail daily. I will e-mail you from time to time, particularly if I encounter a rough patch with emotional eating. I'm counting on you to e-mail me within 24 hours with unconditional support. Please understand that I don't need you to lecture me or chastise me about my eating or exercise habits. Rather, I most need you to listen and let me express my feelings. Your e-mails of understanding and support will help motivate me to stay on track.

Please let me know at your earliest convenience whether you can help me. Thanks so much!

_____ (your name)

My e-mail address: _____

P.S. I am starting Monday, _____ (insert date)

Try this letter when you contact your phone buddies.

Hi Gloria,

I consider you one of my good friends, and I need your help and support. I am committed to losing weight so that I can improve my health. I am using Jorge Cruise's *8 Minutes in the Morning for Real Shapes, Real Sizes* weight-loss program.

According to Jorge, to be successful at losing the weight, I need three "phone buddies." I would be honored if you would act as one of my phone buddies. If you agree, I will call you from time to time, particularly when I feel myself turning to food as a source of comfort. I'm counting on you to listen to my feelings and thoughts and offer your support. Please understand that I don't need you to try to talk me out of eating. I just need you to listen, give me a chance to express my feelings, and offer support. Tell me that it's going to be okay and that you understand what I'm going through.

Please let me know at your earliest convenience whether you can help me. Thanks so much!

_____ (your name)

My phone number: _____

P.S. I am starting Monday, _____ (insert date)

Try this letter when you contact your accountability buddy.

Hi Pat,

I consider you one of my good friends and a healthy role model. I hope you can help me. I am committed to losing weight so that I can improve my health. I am using Jorge Cruise's *8 Minutes in the Morning for Real Shapes, Real Sizes* weight-loss program.

According to Jorge, to be successful at losing the weight, I need an "accountability buddy." I would be honored if you would serve as that buddy. I've chosen you because you are already practicing the healthy habits that I want to incorporate into my life.

If you agree to become my buddy, we will meet or talk on the phone once a week for about 30 minutes. During that conversation, I will talk about my weight-loss goals. I'll also talk about two of my proudest accomplishments from the past week as well as two challenges that I am facing at that time. I hope you will listen, offer your positive support and advice, and help me to face each new week with optimism and energy.

Please let me know at your earliest convenience whether you can help me. Thanks so much!

_____ (your name)

P.S. I am starting Monday, _____ (insert date)

mind your buddy of your original weight, the number of pounds you have lost that week, and the total number of pounds you've lost so far. Next, share with your buddy the two things you are the most proud of that you did during the past week. Then share two things you can do better the following week. Finish by asking for your buddy's positive comments.

Go to your support team list now and write "accountability buddy" next to one name on the list. Then write his or her phone, address, and e-mail information.

Ask for help. Now for the hard part: asking your seven buddies to join your inner team.

Mail each buddy a very special "snail mail" letter along with a

copy of your Power Pledge Poster, your healthy weight page, and your Day in the Future Life of the Future Me essay. Also consider including a copy of this book to help your buddies better understand the program. To help you write your letter, I've included three samples you can use as models. You'll find them on page 53.

step 3

Now you're ready for the last step to eliminating emotional eating with The People Solution. You're ready to expand your inner support network!

expand your buddy team

In Step 2 you identified seven good friends to support you on your way to success. Now we're going to expand and strengthen your support network. Think of your support team as a safety net. The more people you bring on to your team, the more strings you weave into your net, making your safety net that much more able to catch you and hold you up should you fall.

So what are the best ways to expand your buddy team? I recommend you start your own

weekly weight-loss group in your hometown and/or join my online weight-loss club. Let's take a closer look at both of these methods.

Start a weekly weight-loss group. By starting your own weekly weight-loss group in your hometown, you will create a great way to meet new people.

Your local bookstore provides the best meeting spot for your weight-loss group. In fact, some Jorge Cruise weight-loss groups are already active in bookstores around the country. (To find a local Jorge Cruise club in your town or for tips on running a

local meeting, go to www.jorge-cruise.com/localclubs.)

If you don't have an active club in your hometown, you can start your own. It's easy! Meet with the manager of your local bookstore. Show him or her this book and tell him or her you want to start a weight-loss book club. Ask for help with publicity. Suggest that the store might add your meeting to its monthly calendar and put up flyers to help with launching the first meeting. If you start a club, tell me about it by e-mailing me at localclub@jorgecruise.com, and I'll add it to my JorgeCruise.com Web site. Plus, if I am ever in your hometown, I just might stop by one of the meetings!

I have received many e-mails from people who have done this, and it works great. For example,

sharon lawson, edna frizzell, and cheryl mccowan lost 56 collective pounds

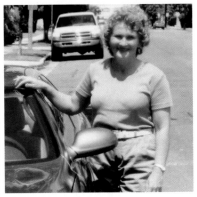

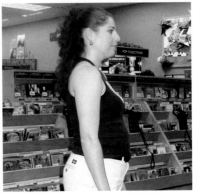

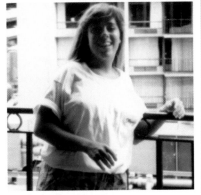

When I joined the Jorge Cruise book group, I met wonderful people like Cheryl and Edna and learned about their weight-loss struggles. Their stories touched my heart.

"Knowing that we all had problems and difficult times made us very supportive of each other."

As we nurtured and cheered each other on week after week, we all felt the power of being part of the group.

You can be a part of a support group via e-mail, phone, or in person. I recommend that everyone find and get support from others, especially while losing weight.

"The extra support helped me lose 23 pounds."

You are not the only one struggling. There are others out there going through the same thing. Hearing other people's stories will help you motivate yourself to move forward toward your dreams. They will be there to listen and guide you along the way.

I met Sharon and Edna at a bookstore. But if you want a virtual place to meet, go to JorgeCruise.com.

"The online support has been incredible."

I look at the Web site as a huge living room where everyone has something in common, and there is always someone around to share anything from recipes and photos to offering a pep talk and guidance. The Web site also gives me the chance to catch up with my buddies Sharon and Edna any night of the week.

The power of the group helped Sharon lose 20 pounds, Edna lose 23 pounds, and Cheryl lose 13 pounds. Don't they look great?

Cheryl McCowan, Edna Frizzell, and Sharon Lawson met at a Jorge Cruise book club at a Borders in San Diego. "I began looking forward to the weekly meetings," Cheryl told me. "It was a place to share and compare what we learned about ourselves during the past week and to process our new insights with each other. Sharon and Edna were in the same pound range as I was, and their excitement and enthusiasm kept me going. They made me feel good and gave me support every step of the way." (Read more about Sharon, Edna, and Cheryl on page 55.)

join the jorgecruise.com online club

You can find a wealth of support at any time simply by going online and letting your fingers do the talking.

I've created numerous chat rooms and discussion areas on my Web site specifically for people just like you. At Jorge-Cruise.com, it does not matter what city you live in, what time of the day it is, or what you are wearing. You just need your computer and a connection to the Internet.

Replacing your trips to the refrigerator with trips to your computer will help fuel your weight loss. Research done at Brown University School of Medicine shows that people who had 24/7 access to interactive support via the Internet lost three times more weight than people who had no interactive online support.

For example, two of my clients, Kim Magaña and Lynnette Perkins, met online at my site and proceeded to inspire each other to lose weight. "Lynnette has been so inspirational to me because of her dedication to the program," said Kim. "It helps me when I am having a weak moment to think about Lynnette and how focused she is. It gets me through that tough spot." (Read more about Kim and Lynnette on page 57.)

With my online club, you will have access to:

- Daily motivational messages from me

- Weekly online meetings

- Live chat auditoriums with myself and others

- Chat rooms for making new friends and buddies

- Expert advice from 8-minute mentors such as Kim and Lynnette

In addition to this wealth of support, you'll also be able to chart your weight loss and much more. Joining our club is like joining a family! That's the power of JorgeCruise.com.

the real solution for real weight loss

By now, I hope you see that you cannot achieve lasting weight loss without first healing your hungry heart. And the only way to heal your hungry heart is by activating The People Solution.

Do not continue reading this book until you have completely finished all of the exercises suggested in this chapter and until you have firmly implemented The People Solution in your life. You wouldn't start a major remodeling job on your house without the proper tools and materials, right? It's the same with completing the three simple steps to The People Solution.

You must have your inner team in place to ensure your success. Be smart, stop reading right now, complete all three steps, and then continue reading this book. Your success at losing weight depends on it.

lynnette perkins and kim magaña
helped each other lose more than 30 pounds each

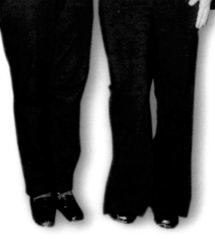

I've lost 33 pounds and 34 inches. I can now bend over without my stomach hurting!

"I can now do things such as putting on pantyhose and tying my shoes without feeling uncomfortable."

There are many people my age, going through menopause, who are really struggling. I feel as if I can be a role model for them. If I can do it, they can too.

With each other's help, Lynnette lost 33 pounds, and Kim lost 30.

I have a very demanding 2-year-old and still have managed to lose 30 pounds! I love the support I get from JorgeCruise.com. That's where I met Lynette.

"Sometimes the little comments I read from people who are losing weight are just what I need to get through a challenging moment in my day or week."

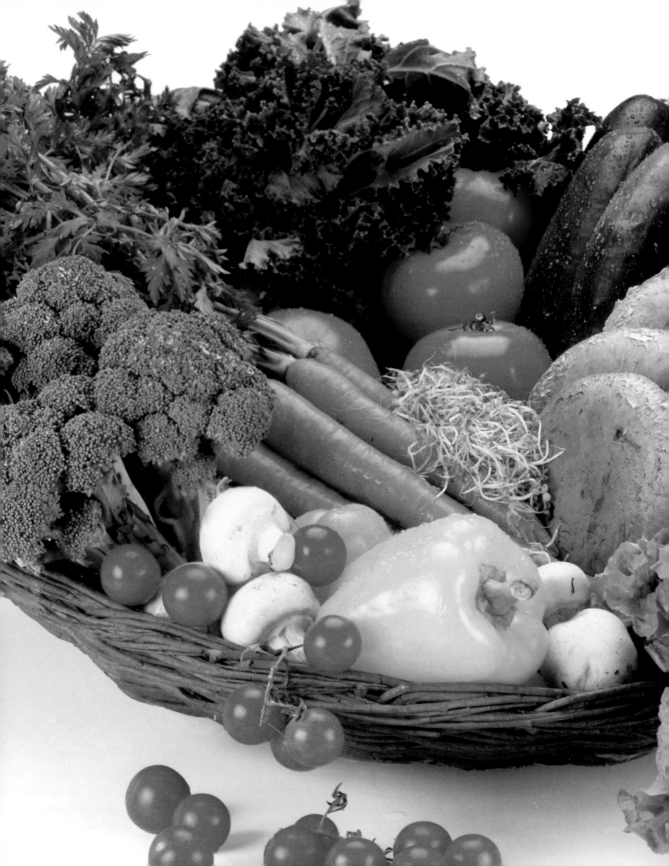

2
How It Works

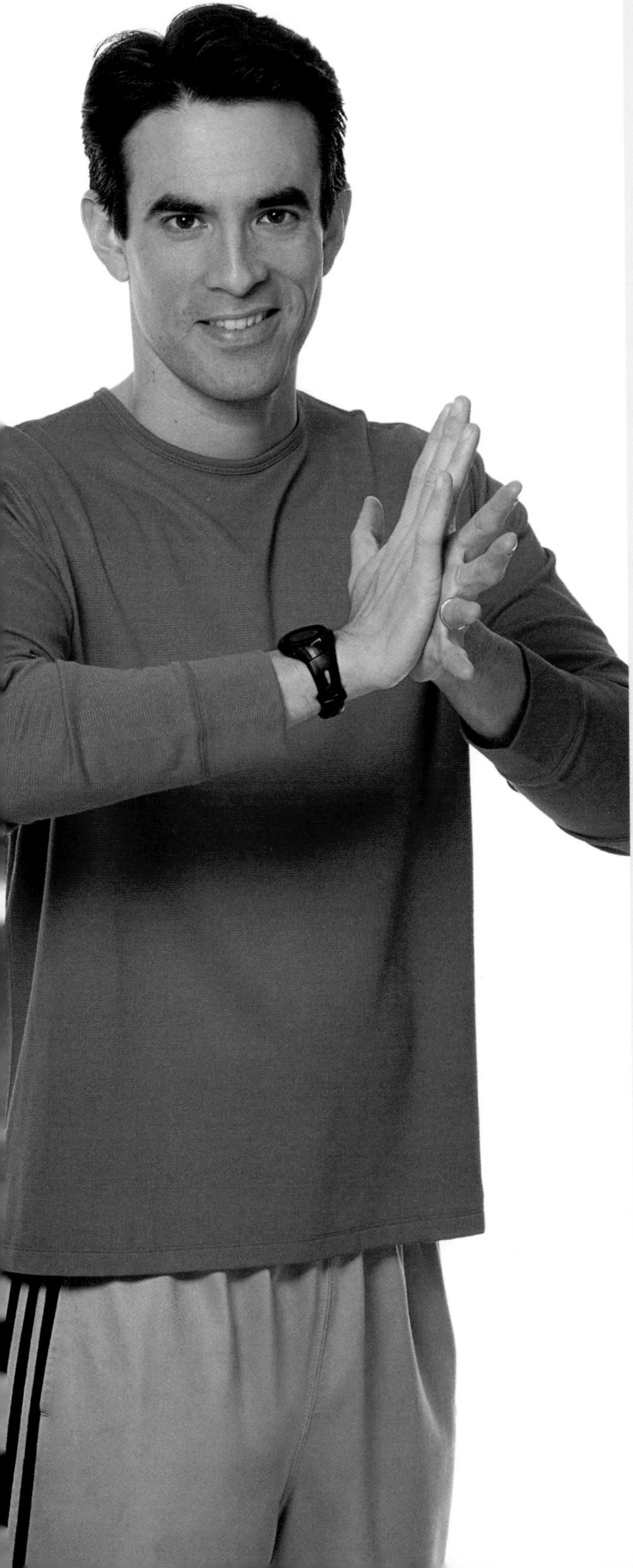

4
Cruise Moves

The 8-Minute
No-Equipment-
Required
Weight-Loss
Secret

how cruise moves burn the fat

When I first met Ann Kirkendall, she claimed she was too busy to exercise. I'll admit, Ann was one of the busiest women I've ever met.

a faithful client shares her story

She was studying to be a school teacher and, at the time, was enrolled in six college courses.

your "8 minute" edge

Once you start using Cruise Moves you will:

1. Dramatically increase your resting metabolism

2. Firm and strengthen your muscles and tighten any sagging skin

3. See major progress in your quest to lose 2 pounds each week

4. Exercise only 8 minutes a day

5. Feel confident about your ability to exercise

6. Enjoy movement, possibly for the first time in your life

Every day she was at school between 7 A.M. and 5:30 P.M. After that, she spent her evening hours doing homework, community service, or observing classes at a local school.

I asked her if she thought she could find just 8 minutes in her day. She said she'd give it a try, so I got her started on my Cruise Moves plan. Now, she's one of my most faithful clients.

"Something magical happens when you dedicate yourself to this program," she said. "I now have more energy. I feel stronger. I've found that I not only have 8 minutes in the morning to do the moves, but more energy all day long. Now, if I ever feel tired and tempted to hit the snooze button in the morning, I remind myself that the moves make me more awake, more alive, and more motivated all day long." (Read more about Ann on page 63.)

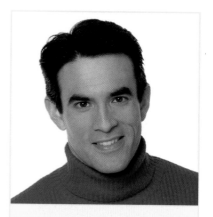

"I'm confident that all the moves that you'll try over the next 4 weeks will work for your body."

Ann is just one of many people who contacted me, asking for a quick-and-easy, effective weight-loss program designed specifically for those who want to lose 30 or more pounds. As I mentioned in chapter 1, when I designed the program for my first weight-loss book, *8 Minutes in the Morning*, I thought I had designed moves that worked for all people, of all shapes and sizes.

I was wrong. Some of the moves were simply too hard or too uncomfortable to perform for those with 30 or more pounds to lose. People wrote to me and complained of back pain or knee pain with certain moves.

But they all also told me they absolutely *loved* the main concepts of *8 Minutes in the Morning*. They wanted a weight-loss program that took just 8 minutes a day, one that they could do in the comfort and privacy of their own homes, one that required little to no equipment, and one that focused on simple, easy-to-learn movements.

The result is my Cruise Moves program. How do I know that this program works for real people of real shapes and real sizes? Because I tested it on people just like you! I'll admit, as with other aspects of my program, I didn't get things perfect the first time around. My faithful and honest testers and clients told me not only when exercises felt too hard or too uncomfortable but also when certain moves seemed difficult to learn and master. Whenever they complained about an exercise, I crossed it off the list and then asked them to try another one in its place.

So I'm confident that all the moves that you'll try over the next 4 weeks will work for your body. They won't hurt. They won't feel uncomfortable. And they won't make you feel clumsy.

But most important, I know that they will help you to lose weight. As a busy, full-figured person, it is critical that you focus on the most effective fat-burning moves that will help ensure your 2-pound-a-week

ann kirkendall lost 35 pounds

For years, my excuse for not getting fit or following a healthful eating plan was that I was too busy. I always felt that I was under too much stress, that whatever time it was, it wasn't the right time to start exercising or eating right. But I learned that there's never a perfect time to make a change, that I just had to do it.

> "There's no better time than now, so get started!"

I also learned that I only needed 8 minutes a day to see amazing results. I now feel amazing. This program works because it is simple and livable and realistic.

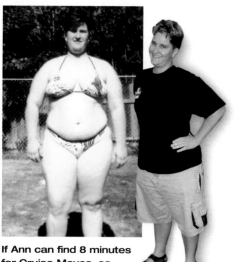

If Ann can find 8 minutes for Cruise Moves, so can you!

weight-loss goal. Welcome to Cruise Moves. I'm confident that you'll *love* the routine. Let's take a closer look.

the science behind cruise moves

So what are Cruise Moves? They are unique strength-training moves that take only 8 minutes a day to complete. What makes them so different and revolutionary? They require absolutely no special equipment, no aerobic activities, and no difficult or hard-impact movements that could hurt your back or joints. Plus, they can be done while wearing your favorite pair of pajamas within the privacy of your own home!

Like other types of strength-training programs, Cruise Moves encourage your body to build muscle. This is so important because more muscle mass is the number one secret to improved fat-burning and weight loss.

You see, the excess fat on your body is *not* the source of your problem. You may not like having excess fat, but that fat is not to blame. It is only the symptom.

The real culprit is a lack of lean muscle tissue, which burns calories 24 hours a day. And the more lean muscle you have, the more fat you will burn throughout the day. Bottom line: *Lean muscle mass is what controls your metabolism.* (More on this a little later.)

But the problem for so many Americans today is that we are using our muscles less and less. Not even a hundred years ago, we kept our muscles in shape by washing clothes by hand, walking most places that we needed to go, gardening without the help of rototillers, and generally using our bodies to accomplish just about everything that needed to be done in life.

The industrial and technological revolutions, however, have introduced one time- and effort-saving device after another, reducing our reliance on our bodies. We now travel while seated in a car, rather than walking or riding a bicycle. We work at desk jobs, rather than out in the fields. We shop at grocery stores, rather than growing our own food. We play games on the computer, rather than outside on a playground with our kids.

Yet, without movement and use, our muscles begin to shrink and wither away. When your muscles start to become flabby, weak, and Jell-O-like, your metabolism comes to a screeching halt. You see, unlike fat, muscle is metabolically active. Each muscle cell contains a calorie-burning compartment that burns fat and sugar to create energy to fuel not only muscle movement but also muscle maintenance. Because your muscles are busily breaking

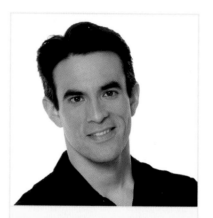

"After just your second or third week on my program, you will feel so energetic and strong that you will find yourself doing things you never thought possible."

down and rebuilding proteins every day, they burn about 50 calories for each pound of muscle.

Researchers estimate that our sedentary lifestyles cause us to actually *lose* 1 to 2 pounds of muscle mass during each decade of life after age 20. By age 50, that means your metabolism may be burning 300 fewer calories a day!

So you see, it's your weakened muscle fibers—and not your fat—that is the true source of your problem. Doing my Cruise Moves will help you reverse this muscle-wasting cycle by building lean muscle that will help you to lose weight and keep it off. It's that simple. The more lean muscle tissue you have, the more body fat you will burn.

Imagine you are a Volkswagen Beetle but that your mechanic has upgraded your engine to a more powerful one from a brand new Porsche. Would this stronger engine consume more fuel? Of course it would. The same is true with strength training. When you create more muscle (a stronger engine), you burn more fat (your stored fuel).

Each pound of muscle revs up your metabolism by up to 50 calories a day. My Cruise Moves will help you firm up 5 pounds of lean muscle within the first few weeks, allowing your body to

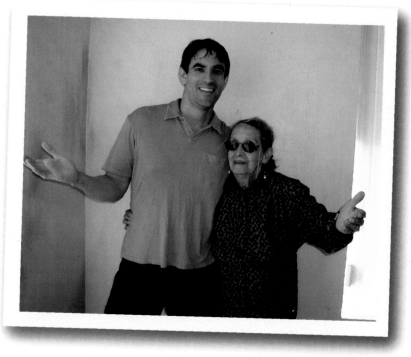

Grandma Maria started strength training when she was 91 years old.

burn an extra 250 calories a day. That amounts to more than 25 pounds of fat each year! The more lean tissue you have, the more body fat you will shed, even at night when you are sleeping. (I love that!)

Normally when you go on a diet, 75 percent of your lost weight comes from fat and 25 percent from muscle. This puts you in a vicious cycle, because each loss in muscle mass slows your metabolism, and you must eat less and less to maintain your weight loss. Eventually you gain it all back—and then some—because your metabolism is slower than before you went on the diet.

But when you combine my Cruise Moves with my delicious Cruise Down Plate, you lose nearly all fat and no muscle. You *will* see results—by an average of 2 pounds a week.

cruise moves work for everyone

Here's even more exciting news. It does not matter how old you are to see results. My grandma Maria, who is 93, started strength training 2 years ago, and today she is more vital, healthy, and vibrant than women half her age. She lives alone, prepares her own meals, and is as strong as an ox! She is my super-*abuelita*!

And grandma Maria is no anomaly. Study after study conducted on people age 70 and older has found that strength training can build lean muscle at any age—literally reversing the muscle-wasting aging process.

If you're a woman, you may be wondering whether strength-training exercises will make you look "big and bulky." Don't worry. Women's bodies don't produce as much of the growth-producing hormone testosterone as men do. Men produce up to 30 times more testosterone. Back in the 1980s, you might

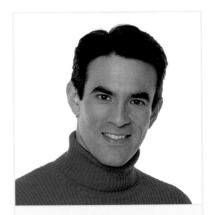

"My program requires only 48 minutes a week to achieve the same amount of muscle building as other programs."

have seen women bodybuilders who looked like men. They followed a very different kind of training program and achieved "he-men" looks with steroid supplements. With my plan, your muscle will only become more firm, sexier, and shapelier—not bulkier.

But you don't have to take my word for it. Here's how Toni White, one of my clients, described her body after doing my Cruise Moves for 8 weeks: "I feel physically stronger. I've lost 12 pounds and already see a difference in how my arms and legs look. I've lost 18 inches in just a couple months. It's magical!"

And the thing you will like even more as time goes by are the antiaging benefits of strength training. According to a study of postmenopausal women, the body becomes 15 to 20 years more youthful after just 1 year of strength training. Other research shows that strength training lowers your blood pressure, cholesterol, and risks for diabetes, heart disease, cancer, osteoporosis, and gastrointestinal problems.

And here's the best news: After just your second or third week on my program, you will feel so energetic and strong that you will find yourself doing things you never thought possible. You will opt to take a walk in the evening instead of sitting in front of the television. You will want to take the stairs at work, and you will get up more often from your desk to take quick walking breaks throughout the workday. You will ignore escalators, elevators, and moving walkways in favor of your own two feet. All this will even further accelerate your results!

your questions

Will a routine ever take me longer than 8 minutes?

Because you do each of the two exercises for exactly 1 minute, and repeat each exercise exactly four times, almost every single workout should last just 8 minutes. I admit, there are just a few sessions that will take you a little longer because you must work each side of your body separately. But on the whole, you'll almost never need more than 8 minutes to finish your routine.

what sets cruise moves apart from other programs

Up until this point, I haven't told you about results that you could probably achieve on numerous types of strength-training programs, whether you wield dumbbells at a gym, sweat through aerobics, use Nautilus machines, or practice power yoga. Why?

how cruise moves differ

Cruise Moves differ from other strength-training programs in three ways.

• They take only 8 minutes a day

• They require absolutely no equipment

• They are specifically designed for your body shape and size

No other program can make those claims. In fact, just about every other strength-training program requires you to spend 30 or more minutes *each* day lifting heavy, and sometimes expensive, equipment in motions that generally don't feel comfortable for someone who has more than 30 pounds to lose.

Let's take a look at how my program works.

the weekly schedule

You may wonder how you can get away with exercising for only 8 minutes a day. Here's how it works.

Each morning you'll do only two Cruise Moves. You'll do two completely different Cruise Moves each day, so by the end of the week you will have exercised and strengthened every muscle in your body. For example, each Monday you'll start out with a move that targets your chest and a move that targets your back. On Tuesdays you'll do a move for your shoulders and one for your abs. On Wednesdays you'll work your triceps and biceps in your upper arms.

It goes on like this through Saturday, when you will have worked every muscle in your body. You'll take Sunday off and then start all over again on Monday with a new set of moves.

Each pair of moves only takes 2 minutes, and you'll repeat each move four times, finishing within 8 minutes. How can you get so much in just 8 minutes? For one, I've strategically paired the moves so that you'll never need to rest between sets. You simply move back and forth between the two exercises suggested for that day, without a rest break, for 8 minutes. As you work one muscle group, the other muscle group rests and recovers. I like to think of this as working smarter and not harder. Believe me, by the time you're done, you'll have completely

the cruise moves schedule

Each week you will work the following muscle groups in this order:

monday: chest and back
tuesday: shoulders and abs
wednesday: triceps and biceps (arms)
thursday: hamstrings and quadriceps (legs)
friday: calves and butt
saturday: inner and outer thighs
sunday: off

worked the targeted muscle groups for that day!

You'll target each muscle group once a week, completely working and fatiguing the area and then giving that particular body area a week to recover.

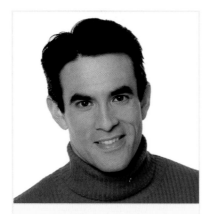

"Before trying my 8 Minutes in the Morning plan, almost all my clients had given up on exercise because other approaches were too difficult for them."

During that week, the muscle fibers in that particular muscle group will build themselves up, becoming firmer, stronger, and more metabolically active.

Other strength-training programs require you to exercise most of the major muscle groups of your body in one very long session, working out every other day to allow the muscles to recover. To me, this is not only a waste of valuable time, but also not the most effective way to burn fat. These programs require you to spend 120 minutes or more at a gym each week, whereas my program requires only 48 minutes a week—to achieve the same amount of muscle building.

Yet, while Cruise Moves may build the same amount of muscle as those other programs, they will actually help you burn many more calories. You see, your body burns calories at a higher rate for 12 to 24 hours *after* a strength-training session. I like to call this the *afterburn* because your metabolic rate skyrockets as your body goes to work repairing and strengthening your muscles. Because you'll do Cruise Moves 6 days out of the week rather than a mere 3 or 4 days required by other programs, you maximize your afterburn, revving up your metabolic rate nearly every day of the week!

Here's how one of my clients, Melissa Farmer, described her results from Cruise Moves: "I never would have believed that 8 minutes of exercising would accomplish anything," she said. "But just in the first few weeks of the program, I was amazed at the muscle tone that started to develop. I always thought you had to work out for hours on the weight machines and strain yourself to get results. Boy, was I wrong! I'm thrilled with how my muscles have started to firm up. My biceps, calves, and thighs especially have responded incredibly well to my Cruise Moves."

Here's what another client, Renee Volz, had to say about Cruise Moves: "I used to work out at least one hour a day and I couldn't lose weight," she told me. "Now, with Cruise Moves, I actually feel stronger, more fit, and most important, am finally seeing results."

no equipment

Here's what truly sets Cruise Moves apart from other strength-training programs, including the program I developed for my first weight-loss book. Cruise Moves require absolutely no exercise equipment! There's no need to find a room in your house to store a weight bench, set of dumbbells, or other equipment. There's no need to buy

maria hoelck lost 42 pounds

I now have muscle definition all over my body, even in places where I didn't know I had muscles! I have strong, firm arms and legs. Even my family life has improved.

> "Keeping up with my kids is so much easier now."

I can run at the park with my son and play tennis with my husband without wimping out. Everyone who has seen me lately notices the difference—and I feel great! I can fit into clothes I wore in college. That thought—that I am as small as I was in college 30 years ago—makes me feel that much younger.

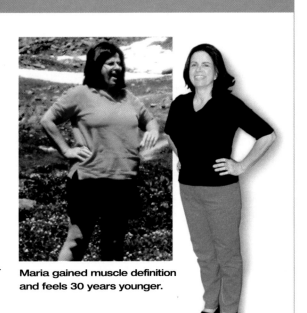

Maria gained muscle definition and feels 30 years younger.

anything. This book is all you need.

My Cruise Moves use unique and proven "holding" and "pumping" motions. I developed these motions with the help and feedback of my 3 million online clients. Bottom line: Each Cruise Move requires you either to "hold a movement" or "pump through a movement." That's it! The only weight you will use will come from your own body. For support, you will sometimes need to use a chair, table, or simple household items like phone books—all simple things that you can find in your home!

These movements are specifically designed to firm and shape your muscles without adding unwanted bulk. No machines, no gyms, and no dumbbells! Of course, if you want to do your Cruise Moves at a gym for variety, you can. And when you're ready to increase the difficulty level, you can move on to my original book, *8 Minutes in the Morning.*

timing is everything

Here's something else that sets Cruise Moves apart. Many other strength-training programs require you to count repetitions, suggesting that you lift a weight 12 to 15 times.

For Cruise Moves, instead of counting repetitions, you will simply watch the clock. You either hold or pump through the suggested Cruise Move for up to 1 minute, and then move on to the next Cruise Move. This frees your mind from counting and forces you to fully fatigue the muscle you are working. It's simple. It's convenient. You'll love it.

I've found with much trial and error in testing this program on my clients that 60 seconds is the ideal amount of time needed to start firming your muscles. In testing this program on client after client, I haven't found a single person who needed to do a move for a longer period of time.

I did encounter some clients,

however, who needed to work up to 60 seconds. If you experience trouble holding or pumping for 60 seconds, that's okay. Start with 30 to 45 seconds and work up to 60 as you get stronger.

designed specifically for you

My challenge to you right now is that you commit yourself 100 percent to using Cruise Moves for the next 28 days. I know you'll love them so much that you will continue to use them until you have lost all the weight you need. Simply follow the plan I have laid out starting in chapter 7 and you will be set!

And don't forget the life-changing results that will come from using Cruise Moves. First, you will dramatically increase your resting metabolism, which means you will start burning fat when you are sleeping. Second, you will firm all weak muscles and prevent sagging skin syndrome. Perhaps most important, you will see major progress in your quest to lose 2 pounds each week in only 8 minutes a day!

your questions

What happens if the Cruise Moves eventually get too easy?

If you feel you need more of a challenge after working through the exercises in chapter 7, then check out my dumbbell routine described in my first book, *8 Minutes in the Morning*.

5
Roll Out of Bed to a New You

Move in the Morning and Lose More Weight

maximize your weight loss

Many people ask me why I recommend so strongly that they exercise in the morning. My answer is always the same. There is no better time than the morning to maximize your weight-loss results with your Cruise Moves.

move in the morning

In the following pages, you'll find out why it's better to get up and move in the morning. You'll also find out proven ways to take advantage of the morning and make it your preferred weight-loss time, even if you think you are *not* a morning person.

That's right. You might be thinking that you are not a morning person. I can hear some of you saying, "Jorge, that will never work for me. As soon as the alarm goes off, I'll hit the snooze button."

Well, I truly believe that there's no such thing as not being a morning person. I know this in part because I used to be a victim of the same belief.

I used to stay up late at night because I told myself that I was a *night person*. I would read, watch TV, and talk on the phone into the morning's wee hours. It's no wonder I always felt tired when my alarm went off in the morning. I never got enough sleep!

When I first tried to exercise in the morning, I thought the task was an impossibility. "Maybe morning exercise works for some people," I told myself, "but it certainly doesn't work for me." But a funny

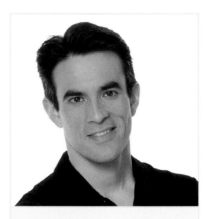

"When I first tried to exercise in the morning, I thought the task was an impossibility."

thing happened along the way. Each time I managed to actually get out of bed and exercise in the morning, I noticed that I felt wonderful for the rest of the day. As time wore on, I was able to get up earlier and earlier. I also felt sleepy

your "8 minute" edge

By exercising in the morning you will:

1. Dramatically boost your metabolism

2. Experience an endorphin high that will make you feel great

3. Ensure you consistently lose 2 pounds a week

earlier in the evening and naturally began going to bed earlier. I stopped being a night owl without really thinking about it.

These days, I never stay up later than 10 P.M., and I'm always out of bed by 6 A.M.

But don't just take my word for it. My clients have all made the same switch. For example, Richard Cross used to get up so late that he spent his mornings in a rush: showering, dressing, grabbing his daily planner, and racing out the door for work. His breakfast—if he ate at all—consisted of fast food he grabbed on the way to work.

His day was then packed with meetings. He usually ate lunch while working at his desk or while talking on his cell phone. After his official workday, he'd head over to a local university to teach a graduate course. Then he'd head home to meet with more clients. He didn't always eat dinner before falling into bed for a few hours of shut-eye before starting it all over again.

But all that changed after he suffered a heart attack. He began to view his body as a car. He decided to treat his old "car" like a new "car." He made his body a priority and then, suddenly, his entire routine changed and fell into place.

"The best time to fix up the old car [your health] is now," said Richard. "If you don't fix it, it will eventually stop working. To paraphrase an old saying, 'Of all the wealth in the world, your health is the most precious.'" (Read more of his story below.)

So you see, if Richard can do it, I *know* you can do it. You'll soon read about proven ways to help easily change your body clock from a night owl to a morning person. But first, let's take a look at why morning exercise is so good for you.

richard cross lost 44 pounds

Jorge's plan helped me focus and understand that my body is like a car. If you do not maintain the car, it will eventually quit working. That's what happened to me.

"I had a heart attack as a result of my poor food and exercise habits."

Now that I have lost 44 pounds, I no longer wonder if there will be another heart attack. There won't. Now I have more energy. I jog up stairs and ride more than 30 miles each week on my bike. I'm actually less hungry now that I am following the program. Best of all, it only requires 8 minutes of my time, a small investment to keep my body running efficiently.

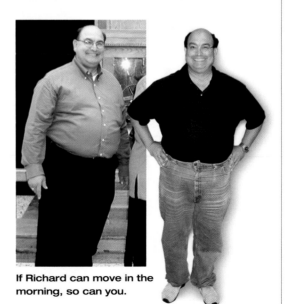

If Richard can move in the morning, so can you.

morning metabolism miracles

Here's some more proof to convince you to try morning exercise. When you first wake up, your metabolism is sluggish because it has slowed down during sleep. But when you exercise, your metabolism increases.

By doing your Cruise Moves first thing in the morning, therefore, you dramatically enhance your metabolism when it's normally the slowest. The bottom line is that physiologically, you burn more calories when you exercise in the morning, making better use of your exercise time.

The morning is also the time of the day that is the easiest to control. Later in the day, distractions will come up. Your spouse, your children, your job, or an emergency will interrupt your plans and force you to put your Cruise Moves on hold. For example, you may have planned to do your exercise during a lunch break, but a friend then asks you to have lunch. You think, "Okay, I'll do it later." But then after work, your 10-year-old asks for your help with her homework. Then your husband wants to snuggle on the coach. You get the picture.

One study I share with all my clients is from the Mollen Clinic in Phoenix. There, they studied 500 people and found that only 25 percent of evening exercisers consistently did their exercise routines, compared to 75 percent of morning exercisers.

The bottom line is that when you commit to exercising in the morning, you bypass excuses and shed the pounds faster because you are more consistent. The Mollen Clinic's founder, Art Mollen, D.O., explained, "As the day goes on, people pull out the bows and arrows and hunt for excuses not to exercise—like having to work a bit later, run errands, or go out with friends."

Here's another reason to move in the morning: better moods. In a study at the University of Leeds in England, researchers found that women who exercised in the morning reported less tension and greater feelings of contentment for the rest of the day than those who didn't exercise in the morning. When you exercise, you send a signal to your pi-

Enhanced Metabolic Rate

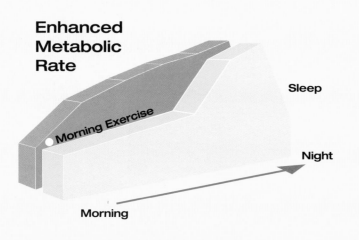

Though your metabolism naturally spikes sometime after midday, exercising first thing in the morning will increase it immediately so that you can reap the benefits all day long.

tuitary gland to release endorphins, your body's natural feel-good chemicals. The more endorphins you have in your bloodstream, the better you feel. Thanks to morning exercise, you will be able to better handle stress no matter what happens in your day, whether it's getting stuck in a traffic jam, dealing with annoying coworkers, or tending to a sick child. Stress will seem to disappear!

And less stress and better moods equal better eating habits. "By exercising first thing in the morning, I make better food choices all day long," one of my clients, Robin Morris, told me. "I now rarely drink soda or eat junk food. As a result, I no longer go to bed feeling like a failure, but instead I feel excited for a new day. Talk about starting the day with a positive step!" (See her photo on page 218.)

And there are still more benefits to exercising in the morning. There is a wonderful study at Indiana University in Bloomington that suggests that morning workouts reduce blood pressure more than workouts done at other times during the day. In fact, morning exercisers experienced an 8-point drop in systolic pressure (top number) that lasted 11 hours. Their diastolic pressure (bottom number) dropped 6 points for up to 4

hours after exercise. Evening exercisers showed no significant reductions.

Finally, according to the American College of Sports Medicine, some evidence confirms that hormonal responses to strength training are strongest in the morning. Resting levels of testosterone, the body's primary muscle-building hormone, are the highest in the morning. In addition, following a bout of strength training, testosterone elevations are more marked in the morning than compared to the afternoon or early evening. This suggests that the muscle-building potential of strength training may be at its peak before noon.

the weight-loss power of sleep

To fit in your 8 Minutes in the Morning, you may need to get up a little earlier. But that doesn't mean you should rob yourself of 8 or so minutes of sleep. I strongly suggest you go to bed earlier!

Why is sleep so important? Well of course you need enough sleep so you can wake up just a bit earlier to do your Cruise Moves. But perhaps even more compelling is that getting more sleep may accelerate your weight loss. Yes, the right amount of

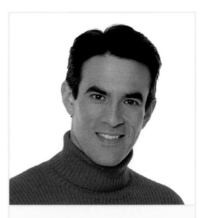

"You burn more body fat when you move in the morning, making better use of your exercise time."

sleep can help you lose more weight.

Let me explain. When you're asleep, your body may shut down many processes; your immune system, however, always works the night shift. While you sleep, your immune system works hard to repair your lean muscle tissues, helping your body to fully recover from the Cruise Moves session that you did in the morning. Growth hormone levels are at their highest during sleep, encouraging your muscles to patch up any microtears and to grow stronger.

Most of us get a least an hour too little sleep on a regular basis. This isn't good. Research has linked getting fewer than 8 hours sleep to the following:

- Poor work performance

- Negative emotions such as anger, stress, sadness, and pessimism

- Impatience and aggravation

- Road rage

- Impaired memory

- Mood swings

And that's only the beginning. One study done in Mexico found that just 1 day of sleep deprivation decreased insulin sensitivity, making it harder for fat and sugar to get into the cells that burn them for energy. Another study done at the University of Chicago found that a week of sleep deprivation chronically

THE POWER OF PREPARATION

All of my clients who have reached their goal and maintained their weight loss long-term used what I call the power of preparation.

They all spend at least 5 extra minutes each day after their morning Cruise Moves to focus on preparing for the rest of their day. They write down a to-do list and schedule their weight loss into their daily calendar.

They literally write down their meals, what they plan to eat, and when they plan to eat them. They flip to the next morning and pencil in their morning exercise session. If they wear special exercise clothing, they get out the next day's clothes and lay them out neatly near the bed. They make their lunch and check to make sure they have the food they need for a healthy dinner.

The whole process can take as little as 5 minutes. But it's a powerful 5 minutes because my clients tell me that the simple process of *writing down* their goals to move in the morning and to eat every 3 hours serves as an incentive to making those goals a reality.

Here's how the power of preparation has worked for one client in particular, Jacqui Poor, a busy television producer. Each night

before bed, she activates the power of preparation by preparing foods that she will eat the next day. She cuts up vegetables, grills or prepares protein, and makes salads. She divides up her snacks and treats into small baggies to take with her.

"The quicker access I have to these foods in the morning, the faster I can start my day," she told me.

Each morning she gets up, reviews her Power Pledge Poster, essay, "before" and "after" photos, and does her Cruise Moves. She eats breakfast, sets out her clothes for the next day's moves, packs up her snacks and lunch for work, and heads out the door. (Read more about Jacqui on the next page.)

If, like Jacqui, your life is busy, I strongly recommend that you stay organized and focused. To help you do this, I have included my Cruise Weight-Loss Planner on page 246. Simply take that master page to any copy store and photocopy enough for the next few months. You will love it!

jacqui poor lost 45 pounds

I used to be afraid to fly on planes because of the narrow aisle and that 5-minute search to find a seat. I could clearly read what was on most of my fellow passengers' minds by the looks in their eyes that said, "Please don't sit next to me." Well, all of that changed.

> "This program is a blessing to me. It has given me a new life."

I have lost 45 pounds! My insecure days of flying are finally over.

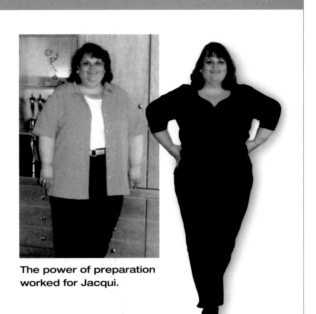

The power of preparation worked for Jacqui.

raised levels of the stress hormone cortisol and brought on a prediabetic state.

Here's more. *Sleep deprivation might even be what's keeping you overweight.* Some studies have linked sleep loss to overeating. Research shows that the later people stay up at night, the more likely they are to overeat. And when you crave late-night munchies, are you really going to reach for something healthful? A study done in Japan found that those who had the fewest hours of sleep tended to eat the fewest amounts of vegetables.

If you get too little sleep, you will snack more during the day, using food to help you stay alert. Lack of sleep also affects your levels of leptin, the hormone that decreases your appetite. When levels are low, you crave sweets and starches. Finally, a study done on men who suffer from sleep apnea—a condition that causes you to stop breathing and wake repeatedly throughout the night—found that fatigue resulting from lost sleep made men less likely to exercise and made exercise feel more difficult.

Getting enough sleep is as important to your overall health as regular exercise and healthful eating. So, promise yourself right now that you will start going to bed earlier. It will help you wake up easier and lose weight faster. It's really important to your success.

your questions

I work the night shift. For me, what most people consider the morning is when I'm winding down to go to bed. My true morning starts around 3 P.M. Is this when I should do my exercises?

Do your exercises as soon as you get out of bed, whatever time of day that is. That's the time of *your* day when you have the most control.

scheduling your 8 minutes in the morning

So now you might be thinking, "Okay, Jorge. I'm convinced. But how do I schedule the time in the morning? I am so busy!"

make time for sleep

Ideally you should rise, review your Power Pledge Poster, go to the bathroom, splash some water on your face, drink a glass of water, and then do your Cruise Moves. Do nothing else before you finish those tasks. That is what I personally do each morning.

Every day I wake naturally at 6 A.M. I no longer need an alarm clock. As long as I consistently go to bed at 10 P.M., I naturally wake up at 6 o'clock.

I keep a copy of my Power Pledge Poster on my bedside table. If I experience the slightest urge to stay in bed, I look it over. I also read my ultimate references that remind me how important my body is. I remember that I'm soon going to be a dad and that I want to be healthy and have energy for my wife and child. I remember that I need to be able to be active in order to train my clients. Finally, I remember that a strong, fit body gives me freedom.

Then I'm out of bed, no problem. I'm off to the bathroom to take care of business, splash some water on my face, and again review the Power Pledge Poster that I have taped to the medicine cabinet.

Then I do my Cruise Moves. Yes, I follow the same exercise program that I suggest for my clients. Ever since I wrote my first book, my life has become busier and busier, and an efficient 8-minute-long exercise plan has become more and more necessary! After I do my moves, I eat breakfast and start my day.

DISCOVER YOUR LOSER ZONES

List your top three loser zones below, along with how much time you spend in each zone per day.

Loser zone activity #1: _____   Minutes per day: _____

Loser zone activity #2: _____   Minutes per day: _____

Loser zone activity #3: _____   Minutes per day: _____

Once you've listed your loser zones, add up all the time spent in them.

Total loser zone time: _____   (NEW potential sleep time!)

I know you can do it, too. Here is my secret for making Cruise Moves happen each morning. We all have what I call a "loser zone," where most of us spend too much time each day. You fall into this loser zone when you spend your time doing things that produce no significant improvement in your life. Watching television ranks as the number one loser zone activity. The average American spends 30 hours a week watching it. Your loser zone might also involve aimlessly chatting on the phone or excessively surfing the Internet.

What are your loser zones? And how many hours a day do you spend per loser zone activity? If your total number per day is more than 1 hour, you have just found some time that you can use to get to bed earlier and therefore wake up a bit earlier to do your Cruise Moves!

To help you determine your loser zones, fill out the "Discover Your Loser Zones" chart on page 78.

Once you determine your loser zones, commit yourself to staying out of them. If you do so, you will create a minimum of 1 more hour each day. Use this hour to get more sleep. Go to bed 1 hour earlier at night. That extra hour of sleep will help to reset your body clock, allowing you to wake up refreshed and rejuvenated and ready to face the Cruise Moves.

more tips for night owls

I know some of you will still experience difficulty getting up in the morning, particularly in the first couple weeks of the program. Some of you are probably muttering to yourselves, "I need all the help I can get!"

That's why I scoured the latest research on sleep as well as asked my clients to send me tips describing what helped *them* get up earlier in the morning. Two of my clients in particular, Regina and Stephan Carey, had a lot to say about morning exercise.

"Finding time to exercise, eat right, or shop for food was extremely difficult before we started the program," they told me. "Now, we have not missed a morning of exercise. If we did, we would feel as if we had forgotten to brush our teeth or take a shower. It has become a way of life that jump-starts our days and provides the energy we need to tackle our daily activities."

Morning movement is so important to them that Stephan and Regina take extra precautions to make sure they get out of bed on time. First, they allow themselves a small luxury of hit-

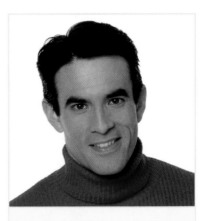

"An extra hour of sleep will help to reset your body clock, allowing you to wake up refreshed and rejuvenated and ready to face the Cruise Moves."

ting the snooze button once—but no more. "My snooze allows me 9 minutes of extra sleep," explained Regina. "I usually spend that time lying in bed thinking of all the things I have to do."

As soon as the alarm rings again, they get up. Their

stephan and regina carey lost more than 60 pounds

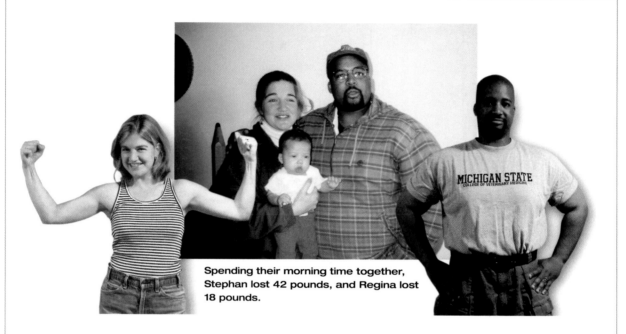

Spending their morning time together, Stephan lost 42 pounds, and Regina lost 18 pounds.

We are a very busy family. With two professional careers, two children, and a dog, we go from one institution to the next—dropping off, picking up, playing sports, attending birthday parties, grocery shopping, doctors' appointments, and so on.

> "Exercising in the morning has changed the way we run our morning routine by carving out personal time each day."

Eight minutes of solitude in the morning is precious, considering the way we spend the other 23 hours and 52 minutes! We have come to rely on this time as a healthy way to start our day.

workout clothes are right next to the bed, where they placed them the night before. As soon as they rise, they get dressed for their workout before leaving the bedroom. The method never fails. (You can read more about Stephan and Regina above.)

Here are some more tips for getting out of bed in the morning.

Believe in yourself. Simply put, if you believe you are a morning person, you will become a morning person. Our thoughts are powerful and con-

trol our actions. Change your thoughts, and your actions will soon follow.

Get up with the sun. Our natural sleep-wake cycles are governed by sunlight. Artificial lighting, however, tends to throw off this natural cycle, allowing us to feel alert at night when the world's natural darkness would otherwise signal our brains to feel sleepy. Artificially darkened rooms also throw off this cycle, making us feel tired in the morning when natural sunlight would otherwise wake us up.

That's why I suggest you get up with the sun. Stop pulling your shades down when you go to bed at night. That way, your room will become lighter and lighter as the sun rises, and you'll already be awake and alert long before your alarm clock sounds. During the winter months, when the sunrise is later, you might invest in a special type of alarm clock that's really a lamp that wakes you up by slowly increasing the amount of light in the room. Sold under the brands Bodyclock and Rise and Shine, among others, you can set these "clocks" for a certain time, and they will slowly illuminate your room, waking you naturally.

Take baby steps. Your body has a set internal clock, so at first, you'll have a hard time falling asleep an hour or more earlier than you're used to. Start by changing your bedtime by just 15 minutes. Then, when you're used to that, add another 15, and then another 15, until you're going to bed an hour earlier.

Wean yourself off caffeine. The more dependent you are on caffeine, the harder it will be for you to wake up in the morning. Try half-caffeine and half-decaf coffee at first. Then, switch to either green tea, which has less caffeine than coffee, or all decaffeinated coffee. Then switch to decaffeinated tea.

Create a sleep sanctuary. If you feel tired during the day but are already getting 8 or more hours of sleep, you're probably not sleeping well. Don't resort to sleeping pills because they'll just make things worse. Instead, try to eliminate what might be keeping you awake. Wear earplugs to eliminate noise. Try taking a warm bath before bed to soothe away stressful thoughts or tension that might be keeping you awake. The warm bath will also raise your body temperature. As your temperature returns to normal after the bath, you will automatically feel sleepy.

Affirm your wake-up time. As I've mentioned before, our minds are extremely powerful motivators. As you fall asleep at night, repeat a positive affirmation to yourself such as, "I will wake up at [insert time]." Say it over and over to yourself silently. This process will both help you fall asleep faster, as the affirmation will become a form of meditation, and prime your body to awaken at the right time.

Keep a list and check it twice. No matter how many steps you take to ensure you get out of bed in the morning, every once in a while you will encounter a morning when you struggle to get out of bed. For those such mornings, I encourage you to keep a copy of your Power Pledge Poster on the table or dresser near your bed. That way, as you lie in bed, you can remind yourself of all the important reasons to get up, such as your health, your energy

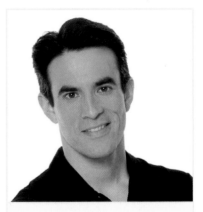

"If you get too little sleep, you will snack more during the day, using food to stay alert."

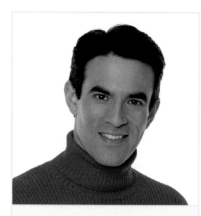

"Try taking a warm bath before bed to soothe away stressful thoughts or tension that might be keeping you awake."

levels, your mood, and your happiness.

Don't give yourself an out. For those of you who really struggle with getting out of bed, I suggest you set two alarm clocks. Place one by your bed and another much farther away, at a place you can only get to if you *get out of bed*. Set them at their maximum volumes so that you can't stand lying in bed while they scream, "Get up and turn me off!"

Get your spouse involved. The times I'm most tempted to linger in bed are the times that Heather is also lingering in bed. There's just something about the presence of a warm body that seems to hold us between the sheets. So to help myself get out of bed earlier each day, I had to ask Heather to help me. Now we both get up at the same time.

Be prepared. If you plan to change into exercise clothing and shoes, always place them by your bed the night before. That way you don't have to think about

getting dressed when you wake up. Also have this book at the ready, opened to the specific day you'll be focusing on.

good morning, sunshine!

So now you see, the morning offers so much weight-loss power. You now know there is no better time than the morning to maximize your weight-loss results with your Cruise Moves.

My personal challenge for you for the next 28 days is to consistently take advantage of the morning and make it your preferred weight-loss time. I know you can do it!

And remember that by doing this you will dramatically boost your metabolism each day. You will also experience an endorphin high that will make you feel great and reduce stress throughout your whole day. And most important, you will ensure that you consistently lose 2 pounds a week!

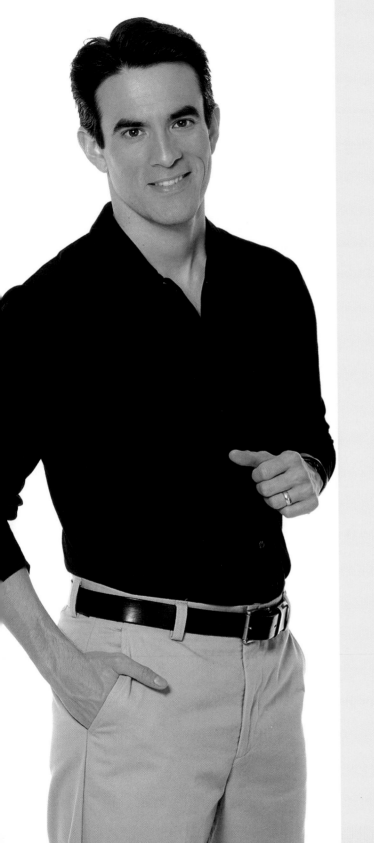

6

The Cruise Down Plate

Bring Back the Joy of Eating without Deprivation, Starvation, or Calorie Counting

enjoy eating once again

Are you ready to bring back the joy of eating? Well, I have exciting news. You can successfully lose weight—more easily—by eating your favorite foods and enjoying every taste.

time for a better way

It may seem counterintuitive, but most people try to lose weight by doing just the opposite. They tell themselves that they can't eat cake, that they need to count calories, skip meals, or generally try to starve off the fat. But those methods always backfire. Sure, they might help you lose weight—at first—but the weight never stays off for long. If you've ever tried to lose weight with such methods, you already know this, and I'm just preaching to the choir.

It's time for a better way, and after much research and trial and error, I've found the answer in the Cruise Down Plate. It's my revolutionary and extremely easy way to lose weight, and I'm convinced that you will love it.

Now, before I share with you the magic of the Cruise Down Plate, I must first tell you why you must never again deprive yourself, starve yourself, or count calories. Those three methods will only keep you at your current weight or even fuel

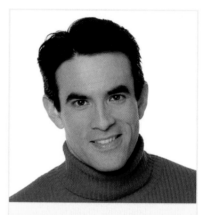

"Even *thinking* about banning foods from your diet can bring on food cravings."

weight gain. Why? They are not practical in real life. Let me explain.

deprivation

Any diet that tells you that you can't eat this food or that food—especially if they are foods you

---

your "8 minute" edge

The Cruise Down Plate allows you to:

1. Eat the foods you love

2. Eat confidently at any restaurant, party, special occasion, or holiday gathering

3. Snack every day on delicious foods, including chocolate!

4. Get the ideal amount of protein to support lean muscle growth.

like—is a depravation diet. For example, some deprivation diets make you give up bread or pasta or dessert or meat. Though such diets can help you to lose weight, they generally fail miserably at helping you to keep the weight off.

Think about it. Giving up bread for 8 weeks may sound doable, but how about a year? Could you give it up for that long? Okay, well, how about the next 50 years? No way!

Humans are hardwired to crave a variety of foods. If you stop eating carbohydrates, or protein, or fat, your body will eventually crave these foods more than ever. Then when you give in, you binge and gorge on the food, eating huge amounts of it that you would have never eaten had you not been on the deprivation diet.

I've heard about this problem over and over again from my clients. For example, one client told me that she had recently lost 15 pounds by giving up cheese, but that the weight had been creeping back because she couldn't seem to find the willpower to stay away from cheese for good. She asked me to help her find the willpower to "stay off the cheese." I told her, "You don't need willpower. You need a realistic eating plan."

I've heard similar stories from many of my online clients. Before they could lose weight—and keep it off—they all had to learn that deprivation usually causes more weight gain in the long-term.

You see, research shows that even *thinking* about banning foods from your diet can bring on food cravings. A study done at the University of Toronto found that students who were told that they were about to embark on a week-long diet that restricted particular foods were more likely to consume more food the night before the "diet" than other students who were not told they would soon start a diet. A different study done at the University of Gainesville in Florida found that students who routinely deprived themselves of certain foods responded to pictures of certain foods with increased heart rates and more sensitive startle reflexes. And finally, another study done at Louisiana State University found that people with the most flexible eating habits were more likely to eat reasonable food portions than those with the most restrained eating habits.

starvation dieting

You may have been told that weight loss is easy . . . just don't eat. And research does show that

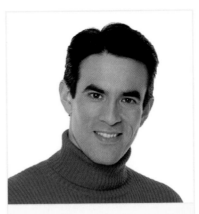

"If you fill up on vegetables, you can literally eat more food— more often— and still lose weight."

you can lose unwanted weight by starving yourself. The problem is that up to 50 percent of that weight comes from muscle tissue loss, not from fat loss. And that sets you up for pure *disaster*.

If you recall from chapter 4, your muscle tissue is your body's metabolic furnace. Every pound of muscle burns up to 50 calories a day. This means that every pound of muscle you lose on a diet slows your metabolism down by 50 calories a day. As your metabolism slows down, you'll have to eat less and less food to compensate.

But it doesn't stop there. As you starve yourself, your body literally goes into starvation mode. It overproduces certain enzymes that tell your fat cells to hold on to fat and underproduces other enzymes that tell those cells to release fat. At the same time, your thyroid gland signals

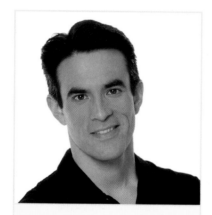

"The Cruise Down Plate will give you the ideal portion of protein to build lean muscles."

your body to *conserve* calories by turning down your overall metabolic rate.

Eventually, weight loss becomes extremely difficult and you hit that all-too-familiar plateau. Few people can continue to eat so few calories for any length of time, and as soon as you start eating normally again, your body will regain the weight you just lost. And because nearly all of that regained weight goes straight to your fat cells, your metabolism will stay just as sluggish. This is why many people who lose weight end up gaining back more than they originally lost.

Also, starvation diets almost always end with a binge. Scientists have shown that even rats and other animals will respond to calorie restriction by binge eating. Other research shows that as soon as people begin a starvation diet, they become preoccupied with food.

Finally, starvation diets are just plain bad for your health. One study done at the University of Carolina at Chapel Hill found that 7 days of a starvation diet resulted in elevated cholesterol levels, particularly the unhealthy LDL cholesterol.

calorie counting

All right, how many times have you tried to write down all of the calories you've eaten in a day? Was it ever easy? No way!

Here is what I have learned from my clients. If a weight control method becomes too difficult and time consuming, you will not stick with it long-term. Think about it. How many books would you have to read to learn the caloric values of foods? How many minutes would you spend reading labels? How long could you keep it up? How much fun would that be? How much time would it drain from your day? I say just forget it. In today's busy world, time is just too precious to be counting the calories of every food you eat.

Few people are able to successfully pull it off, and even fewer are able to keep it up for long. Studies bear this out. One study done at Louisiana State University actually linked calorie counting with overeating!

the cruise down plate

Now that you know what not to do, you're ready to find out what *to do* to lose weight successfully. Enter the Cruise Down Plate eating system. It's an amazingly simple way of eating your breakfast, lunch, and dinner that will transform the rest of your life—and, of course, your waistline.

To get started, you'll need a standard 9-inch dinner plate. For your three main daily meals, mentally divide the plate in half. Fill the upper half with vegetables. Then again mentally split the bottom half of the plate into two equal parts. Fill the left side with a high-protein food and the right side with a carbohydrate food. Finally, add 1 tablespoon of fat to help curb your appetite. (You'll learn more about the wonderful appetite-suppressing effects of fat on page 95.)

If you fill up your plate with those portions and eat everything on your plate—and you're still hungry—you may dish yourself up another plate of vegetables. It's that's simple.

And that's really all you need to know to use my Cruise Down Plate to achieve weight-loss success. Of course, I know there will be some of you out there with many questions. You may wonder how high you can pile the food on your plate. Or, after years of calorie counting, you may not feel confident using such a simple eating method. That's where the Resources section of this book comes in. On pages 232–39, I've included a week of sample Cruise Down Plate meals to help you get started. I've also included food lists containing hundreds of vegetables, carbohydrates, fats, proteins, snacks, and treats along with their corresponding serving sizes. So if you're the type of person who feels more secure knowing the exact food portions, you need only consult my food lists.

No matter how you look at it, whether you use the food lists or you just eyeball your portions on your plate, there's no starvation, no hunger, and no complicated arithmetic! By using my Cruise Down Plate eating system, you get the perfect amount of *protein* to help build your "fat-burning" lean muscle tissue. The Cruise Down Plate will also show you how to continue to eat the foods you love in the *right portions*.

It worked for Bonnie Barrett. The Cruise Down Plate helped her lose 33 pounds. "I'm a highly visual person, so the Cruise Down Plate allows me to simplify my meals and keep the weight off," she told me. "The concept is so easy to grasp and follow. I just have to look at a plate and fill each of four areas with one portion of vegetables, protein, or carbohydrates, and one tablespoon of fat. At first I used a plate that was already divided, but now I can eyeball the right portions, even at restaurants." (Read more about Bonnie on page 88.)

your questions

How high can I fill my plate?

Generally, no more than 1 to 2 inches. To get a specific idea of the right protein, carbohydrate, and fat servings for your plate, check out my food lists in chapter 10. I've done all the math and calculations for you. Think of those lists as training wheels. Spend a week measuring out your food portions, making a mental note as to how much space certain foods take up on your plate. After just 1 week, you'll be able to simply look at your plate—without measuring—and know you're on the right track.

It also worked for Ann Kirkendall, whom you met in chapter 4. "The Cruise Down Plate is a blueprint for portion sizes," she said. "In our world of supersizing, we have become a society with a distorted view of what proper portion sizes actually look like. When you use the Cruise Down Plate, you train your body and your eyes to recognize correct portions."

Besides placing your foods on your plate in the right portions, you'll also follow three additional rules for optimal Cruise Down Plate success:

bonnie barrett lost 33 pounds

Before losing 33 pounds, I was in hiding. Yes, hiding myself in my home, under long matronly dresses, baggy sweat suits, and big blouses with pants that had elastic bands.

"Today I am enjoying a new lifestyle, thanks to the Cruise Down Plate."

I am eating healthy foods that actually help keep my weight from yo-yoing. I am putting on muscle to burn food faster. Out in the real world, I no longer have to struggle to put on a happy face. I am happy and it shows!

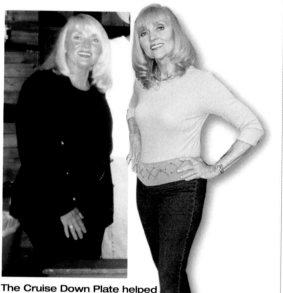

The Cruise Down Plate helped Bonnie drop the weight.

1. You must never skip a meal

2. You must eat two snacks a day

3. You must finish each day by indulging in a delicious treat

Does it sound too good to be true? Many of my clients were just as skeptical when I asked them to test the Cruise Down Plate for me. They told me, "Jorge, I'm trying to lose weight. I cannot eat that many meals and snacks in one day!"

To help ease your fears, here's a little science about why this program works so well. It's all about filling yourself up with low-calorie foods and eating to support muscle growth. With my Cruise Down Plate, half your plate will be filled with vegetables, which are extremely low-calorie foods. For example, an entire cucumber contains only 40 calories, a half-cup of celery only 10 calories, and 10 florets of cauliflower only about 40 calories.

Besides being low-calorie, vegetables are fiber-rich foods that fill up your stomach, which sends the "I'm full" signal to your brain and helps you to feel satisfied all day long. Filling up on vegetables leaves no space for megacalorie foods. Then, one-quarter of your plate is filled with *protein*. Thus, your body is getting the number one material it needs to build lean muscle. And remember, lean muscle equals a faster metabo-

lism. You wouldn't want to waste your 8-minute Cruise Moves by not eating the right amount of protein, would you?

Here's another secret to my Cruise Down Plate: timing. If you eat just one meal a day, skip breakfast, avoid snacks, or deprive yourself of a daily treat, you will actually *slow down* your

plate pointers

While following the Cruise Down Plate, each day you must eat:

• 3 main meals (breakfast, lunch, and dinner)

• 2 sensible snacks

• 1 delicious treat

THE CRUISE DOWN PLATE™

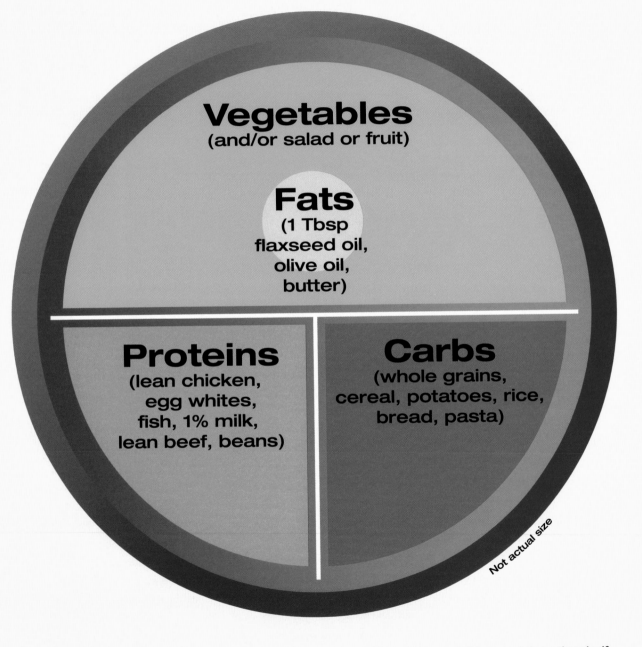

Vegetables
(and/or salad or fruit)

Fats
(1 Tbsp
flaxseed oil,
olive oil,
butter)

Proteins
(lean chicken,
egg whites,
fish, 1% milk,
lean beef, beans)

Carbs
(whole grains,
cereal, potatoes, rice,
bread, pasta)

Not actual size

Follow one simple rule: Fill half of a standard 9-inch plate with vegetables and the other half with equal portions of carbohydrates and protein foods, along with a tablespoon of fat. It's that easy!

A DAY OF EATING WITH THE CRUISE DOWN PLATE

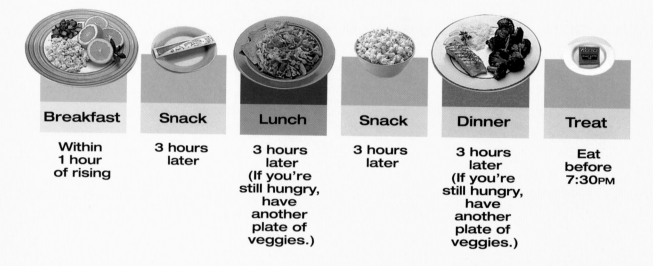

Breakfast	Snack	Lunch	Snack	Dinner	Treat
Within 1 hour of rising	3 hours later	3 hours later (If you're still hungry, have another plate of veggies.)	3 hours later	3 hours later (If you're still hungry, have another plate of veggies.)	Eat before 7:30PM

To see more examples of breakfast, lunch, dinner, snacks, or treats go to pages 233–45.

metabolism, reducing your overall calorie burn and hindering your weight-loss efforts. It's true. Let me explain.

Eating frequent meals in the correct portions is one of the most important things you can do to turn off your body's starvation protection system. Here's how it works. Your body contains a somewhat archaic message relay system left over from our hunting and gathering (and feast or famine) days. This relay system is particularly sensitive to drops in caloric intake. Whenever you go too long without food, this starvation protection

system kicks in. Peptides in your stomach send the message to your brain, which sends the message to various hormonal centers in your body to turn down your body's caloric thermostat. Certain enzymes tell your fat cells to close and lock their doors, essentially only letting calories *in* but not letting them *out*.

End result: You burn fewer calories to accomplish everyday tasks such as moving, breathing, and even exercising. Consequently, your body stores a higher percentage of the food you eat as body fat and only burns off a very small amount for energy.

Worse, when this starvation protection system becomes active, your body must still use calories to survive. Since your body fat is being protected, your body instead breaks down your *lean muscle tissue* as its energy source. This is terrible! As I've already explained, anytime you lose lean muscle tissue, you chip away at your metabolism.

This is why eating frequently—every 3 hours—is so important. It helps to keep that starvation system turned off and your metabolism turned on. Eating frequently makes your stomach and intestines continue to work all day long to break down and digest your food. This, too, increases your metabolism. In essence, the regular supply of calories throughout the day turns up your metabolic furnace, encouraging your body to waste calories and convert them into heat!

To make the Cruise Down Plate timing awareness system work for you, you must follow three simple rules:

1. Eat breakfast within 1 hour of rising

2. Eat every 3 hours

3. Stop eating by 7:30 P.M.

Let's take a closer look at each of these important rules.

eat breakfast within 1 hour of rising

To keep your metabolism running strong, you must eat your first meal within 1 hour of rising. *This is critical.*

As you sleep, your body is not getting any food and consequently turns down your metabolism. This is part of the natural ebb and flow of life, and there's no point in setting an alarm every 3 hours during the night to wake up and eat a snack.

When you awake, however, you want to kick your metabolism back into high gear as soon as possible. If you don't eat within 1 hour of waking, your starvation protection system

will kick in. And when that happens, your body will protect the most precious calorie-rich tissue in your body that it will need to survive during a famine: body fat.

So, you just end up hurting your efforts. The solution is to eat within 1 hour of waking up so that you move your metabolism to the highest possible fat-burning speed. That is why breakfast is so important to your weight-loss success!

eat every 3 hours

Now that you've kicked your metabolism into high gear, keep it that way all day long by eating every 3 hours.

This will help keep that starvation protection system from being activated during the day. The key is eating five minimeals throughout the day separated by 3 hours. In other words, this means you might eat breakfast at 7 A.M., then have a snack at 10 A.M., then eat lunch at 1 P.M., then a snack at 4 P.M., and finally dinner with a treat at 7 P.M. This is a perfect eating schedule, and I strongly recommend you follow it closely.

Snacking will do more than help you lose weight. Some research shows that it may also help lower cholesterol levels. So eat every 3 hours. It's important to your health.

stop eating by 7:30 P.M.

Ideally, you should eat your last meal at or before 7 P.M. and finish that meal—including dessert—by 7:30.

The reason for this is that physiologically, when the sun goes down each day, your body's temperature begins to drop, and vital functions like heartbeat and breathing begin to slow down, readying you for sleep. If you can eat in a way that supports this

your questions

What about foods that combine food groups, such as lasagna, casseroles, and soup?

Always fill half your plate with vegetables first, even if your casserole or other type of dish contains some vegetables. Then, know that your casserole, soup, or other dish can take up no more than half of the rest of your plate. Allow it to count for your carbohydrate and your protein serving (if it contains both). For example, if you are eating tuna-noodle casserole, fill half your plate with the casserole and the other half with a green salad or other type of vegetable.

natural rhythm, you will ensure that your body gets a full night's rest.

Remember in chapter 4 where I told you that the only time your muscles recuperate and get firmer is when you are sleeping? If you eat past 7:30 P.M., you take too much food to bed with you, and your digestive system keeps you awake as it breaks down your food. Though you may actually be able to fall asleep, you won't sleep deeply as your body digests. And you need *deep* sleep in order for your body to truly rest and recover.

If you eat too late at night, your body spends its energy on digestion rather than on repairing and firming your lean muscle tissues. Your goal is to make sure that you recuperate during sleep rather than waste your rest on digestion. I promise you will feel more energized and alive when you wake!

smart eating strategies

Now that you understand how to place food on your plate and how often to eat, let's take a closer look at each of your basic food categories: vegetables/fruit, proteins, carbohydrates, and fats.

vegetables

Vegetables are very important because they are an excellent source of the vitamins and minerals you need for good health. Most exciting for weight loss, vegetables are so low in calories and full of wonderful fiber that

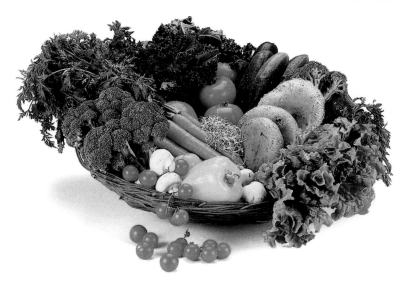

they will keep you filled up longer and never expand your waistline!

Vegetables such as lettuce, cucumbers, broccoli, and sprouts have a very high water content, which means that they are also very high in oxygen. In order for your lean muscle tissue to burn fat, it needs oxygen to help convert the fat into energy. When you eat vegetables, you will flood your body with water, which will dramatically increase your oxygen levels, improving your metabolism.

Second, vegetables are high in fiber, and, ounce for ounce, rank as the most filling low-calorie foods you can eat. Since you must chew vegetables (unlike softer foods such as yogurt), they take longer to eat, allowing your brain the time it needs to turn off your hunger switch. And, of course, once in your stomach, that fiber takes up a lot of space and digests slowly, making you feel fuller for a longer period of time.

Most vegetables are also very low in simple sugars, which is what makes them very low in calories. This means you can literally eat them to your heart's content and not put on excess body fat.

Finally, vegetables are superfoods when it comes down to living a longer life. They provide important vitamins and minerals for your health and energy. Research shows that brightly colored vegetables contain substances called phytochemicals. These phytochemicals help to keep your immune system strong. In just one serving of green, yellow, orange, or red vegetables, you consume as many as 100 different phytochemicals that help to prevent disease. Think about it. If you are sick less often, you will have more time and energy to do your Cruise Moves each day!

fruits

And before I forget . . . let's quickly talk about fruits. Fruits contain the same fiber and important phytochemicals as vegetables. Unfortunately, most fruits also contain more sugar, upping their calorie content.

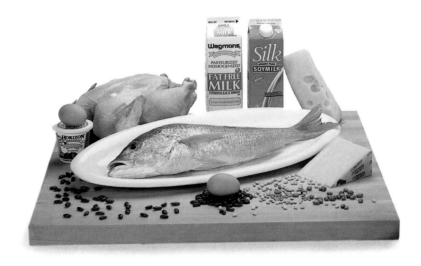

Some fruits also contain simple sugars that your body breaks down too quickly, spiking your insulin levels and preventing you from burning body fat.

That's why I suggest that as you lose weight, hold yourself to eating fruit just once a day, preferably at breakfast. Make vegetables your choice for lunch and dinner. (Once you reach your goal weight, you may add more fruit servings. Consult chapter 8 to find out how.) Lemons and limes are the exception. Feel free to use them as much as you want. (I love to use lemon or lime wedges in my water to make it taste zesty!)

For a full list of all the veggies and fruits I recommend you eat, please refer to my Cruise Down Plate food lists on pages 242–43.

proteins

Protein is the material your body uses to create and maintain lean muscle tissue. More than half your body weight is made up of protein. This includes not only your muscle tissue but also your hair, skin, nails, blood, hormones, enzymes, brain cells, and much more.

When you don't consume enough protein, your body breaks down and recycles existing protein from your lean muscle fibers in order to create protein to fuel essential bodily processes, like your immune system. When this happens, you sacrifice muscle (your fat-burning machine), and your metabolism slows down. As a result, you burn less body fat.

Too much protein, however, is as bad as too little. When you consume too much protein (and as a result, too little carbohydrate), your body burns the excess for fuel. But protein is designed to be a building material, not an energy source, so when you follow a superhigh-protein diet, you end up forcing your body to use protein as a fuel. Unfortunately, protein is a "dirty" source of fuel because it contains nitrogen. Instead of producing just carbon dioxide and water, protein produces toxic byproducts. Your body must pump lots of water into your urinary tract to flush the toxic nitrogen out. In other words, much of the "weight loss" from high-protein diets is simply water loss. While this is going on, you are also losing minerals from your body, including calcium from your bones.

The Cruise Down Plate will help you to automatically eat the right amount of protein to keep your muscles firm and strong. Optimally, you want to choose lean protein foods that are low in saturated (animal) fat. This type of fat adds unwanted calories to your meal, as well as clogs your arteries.

Lean protein foods include egg whites, white-meat poultry, fish, skim or 1 percent milk (or soy milk), low-fat yogurt, and legumes such as beans and lentils. Those are some of the leanest sources available. Try to avoid the proteins high in saturated fat because they will only hinder your weight-loss efforts. When you have a hankering for red meat, go ahead and have it, but choose lean sirloin or round cuts if you can.

For a full list of all the protein sources I recommend you eat, please refer to my Cruise Down Plate food lists on pages 240–41.

carbohydrates

Carbohydrates provide your body with the lighter fluid needed to help burn your stored body fat. Yes, you read that correctly!

Carbohydrates can play a critical role in achieving fat loss. But not just any carbohydrate will help you burn fat. Carbohydrates fall into two categories: whole and refined. You want to consume "whole" carbohydrates when possible. Whole foods have not been overly processed, refined, or bleached. Things like whole-grain bread, whole wheat bread, whole grains like oats, and brown rice fall into the whole foods category.

On the other hand, many types of carbohydrates are *refined*. To make them cook faster, the food industry has peeled off their outer layers and sometimes even pulverized them into smaller pieces. This strips them of their fiber content and makes them digest more quickly. Refined carbohydrates include white bread and rice, instant hot cereals, and low-fiber, sugary breakfast cereals.

Why are whole carbohydrates better for weight loss? They con-

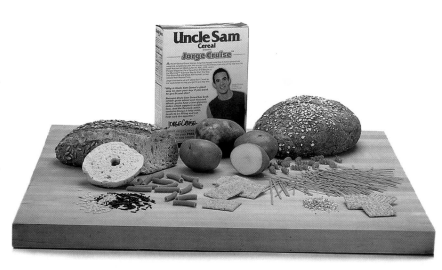

tain more fiber. The more fiber a carbohydrate food contains, the slower it digests and turns into sugar in your bloodstream. The slower a sugar is released into your bloodstream, the more it works like a lighter fluid to burn body fat.

Let me give you an example. Imagine you are starting a campfire. To start burning the logs (your body fat), you would light the big logs by using kindling and a bit of lighter fluid. That is exactly how whole carbohydrates work in your body. Whole carbohydrates supply the lighter fluid you need to maximize your fat burning (the logs). By trickling in small amounts of carbohydrate, your body will burn fat steadily for a long time. But if you were to pour too much lighter fluid (simple, refined carbohydrates) on at one time, you get a flash fire that flares quickly and then burns out almost immediately. That is not the goal.

Unlike refined carbohydrates, whole carbohydrates are not rapidly released into your bloodstream because of their complex molecular structure. This means that whole carbohydrates never overwhelm your body with sugar rushes (or too much lighter fluid) because they take more time to break down. They provide the ideal amounts of *time-released*

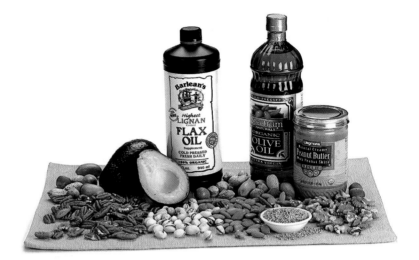

sugar to burn fat. That allows your body to use body fat as its primary fuel.

My favorite kind of whole carbohydrates are whole grains. Whole grains contain their outer shells and are more complex than refined grains, which have been stripped of their outer coatings. In other words, slow-cooking whole grains are better than instant oats, brown rice is better than white rice, whole-grain bread is better than white bread, and whole-grain pasta is better than regular enriched pasta. (One good trick is to check the fiber content on the nutrition facts label of packaged foods. Foods that are higher in fiber, with at least 3 or more grams, tend to be more whole than foods that lack fiber.)

And don't worry if you can't *always* eat whole carbohydrates. Just do your very best to minimize the refined ones, and make every effort you can to eat the whole ones. You will do great!

For a full list of all the whole carbohydrate sources I recommend you eat, please refer to my Cruise Down Plate food lists on pages 241–42.

fats

For years we've been told the best way to lose weight is to eat "fat-free" foods and eliminate as much fat as possible from our diets. Magazine articles, food marketers, and even other weight-loss specialists have told us that all fats are bad and that eating any type of fat will make you fat. Nothing could be further from the truth.

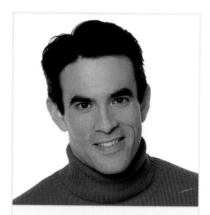

"Flaxseed oil will bring back the joy of eating. It's my favorite type of fat."

You see, not all fats are created equal. Some, such as the omega fats in fish, are extremely good for you and help you shed weight, whereas others, such as the saturated fats in animal products and the "trans" fats in processed foods, are extremely bad for you and also pack on the pounds.

The best types of fats are "omega" fats: omega-3, 6, and 9. Natural foods such as fatty fish, nuts, olive oil, soybeans, flaxseeds and other seeds and nuts, peanut butter, olives, and avocados all contain these important fats. Omega fats will suppress your appetite, promote fat burning, and boost your metabolic rate. They're also extremely good for your health, as study after study has linked these fats with a lower risk for heart disease and certain cancers.

Of the three types of omega fats, researchers suspect omega 3-fats (found in fish, flax seeds, and some vegetables) are the most important for health, longevity, and weight loss.

For a full list of all the good fat sources I recommend you use, please refer to my Cruise Down Plate food lists on pages 243–44.

flax

An example of an omega-3 fat is derived from flax seeds. Flaxseed oil is really amazing. It will bring back the joy of eating to your meals. It's my favorite type of fat.

Here's why. Flaxseed oil is the richest source of the most essential omega-3 fatty acids, important heart-protective fats that help to curb your appetite and prevent fat storage on your body. Omega-3 fatty acids (as well as a few other types of fat) cause the stomach to retain food for a longer period of time as compared to no-fat or low-fat foods. That's because fats require greater digestive energy than proteins and carbohydrates. As a result, they are held in the stomach longer than other food sources, and they help to stimulate the release of cholecystokinin, a gut hormone that signals the brain to stop eating.

But here is the most amazing thing about flaxseed oil: It dose not get stored as body fat!

Your body uses flaxseed oil's omega-3 fatty acids to help maintain the integrity and function of your body's 75 trillion cell membranes to support healthy joints, skin, hair, and strong nails. Because your body uses it for all these reasons, flaxseed oil never gets stored as body fat. No other fat on the planet is that loved or used by your body.

Plus, according to studies done at Pennsylvania State and Thomas Jefferson Universities, of all the nutrients you can eat, the omega fats found in flaxseed oil do the best job of promoting the feeling of fullness and satiety. In other words, you require smaller meals to make you feel satisfied, and you stay satisfied for longer periods of time.

As one of my clients, Sabrina Hahnlein put it, "I live for flaxseed oil. It tastes great and makes my food stick to my ribs. When I eat flax, I'm full, and the feeling of fullness lasts longer. I use it on my eggs every morning, on toast, over steamed vegetables, mixed into pasta, and instead of butter on a baked potato." (Read more about Sabrina below.)

She's not the only one excited about flaxseed oil. Remember Regina Carey from chapter 5? She told me that she uses flaxseed oil to curb any midday cravings. She mixes it into a small container of yogurt for a snack. "It gives me a 3- to 4-hour boost so I can focus on the rest of my life, and not on how hungry I feel," she said.

But that's not all. Flax does more than suppress appetite. Your body uses flaxseed oil to activate your brown body fat, which lies deep within your body and surrounds your vital organs. A leftover from the days when we used to live outside with little clothing to warm us, brown fat wastes calories and turns them into heat. Babies have a lot of this type of fat, which is why they always feel so warm when you hold them, and why they seem to enjoy being naked much more than us adults! So, when you activate your brown fat, you burn more calories and boost your body's metabolic rate.

Finally, flax is also great for your overall health. Research shows that people who consume more flax tend to have lower bad cholesterol levels. Erin McLeod, one of my clients whom you met in chapter 1, lowered her cholesterol from 260 to 165 after she began using flaxseed oil. But that's not all. Another of my clients who lives in a dry climate told me that her skin became softer, smoother, and less itchy once she began eating more flax. It's truly a miracle food!

As I mentioned, flaxseed oil comes from flax seeds, also called linseeds. I recommend that you buy flax in liquid form because it is the most concentrated form

sabrina hahnlein lost 46 pounds

I used to be in a place where *I* didn't matter. My needs and wants never mattered. I wasn't happy with myself and I had no energy. I was achy and miserable. I was only 43 but I felt age 83.

"Now that I have lost 46 pounds, I feel excited about my life."

I need all new clothes because everything I own hangs on me. My energy level is incredible. I wake up every morning feeling awesome. I work my way through the day, and I come home and still feel like I can conquer the world. I ride my bike, play games with my kids, and even run the dog at the beach.

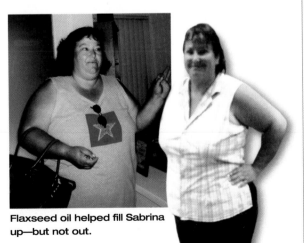

Flaxseed oil helped fill Sabrina up—but not out.

available. The oil is made by cold-pressing thousands of seeds to extract the oil and then is immediately refrigerated to preserve its freshness.

Use the liquid form directly on your foods. Think of it as a great flavor-enhancing condiment you can use with all your meals. I use it during breakfast on toast. At lunch, I put it on my salad, and at dinner, I use it over brown rice or steamed vegetables. Just make sure to not cook with it, as this type of oil doesn't withstand heat very well. Instead, use extra-virgin olive oil or PAM for cooking.

You'll find flaxseed oil in health food stores and some grocery stores. And for those of you who travel or just don't care for the taste of fat, you can get flaxseed oil in capsule form, too.

I am such a big believer in the weight-loss power of flax that I wanted to make sure that all my clients would be able to conveniently find the freshest and finest grade of flax possible at the best price. So I created my own brand of liquid flaxseed oil and capsules, synergized with a proprietary blend of enzymes and antioxidants. It's called Cruise Down Flax Oil. (For more information on Cruise Down Flax Oil, see page 248 or visit www.jorgecruise.com/flax.)

snacks

Each day, you will depend on two sensible snacks to keep your metabolism active and to prevent your starvation protection system from turning itself on. Eat your first snack 3 hours after

breakfast and the second one 3 hours after lunch.

Your snacks also provide a chance for you to indulge a little. As long as you hold yourself to a 100-calorie serving (consult my foods lists on page 244 for some suggested foods at the right serving sizes), you can't go wrong. Of course,

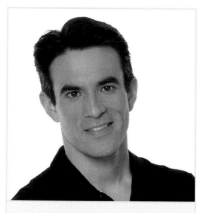

"Eat within 1 hour of waking up and you will move your metabolism to the highest possible fat-burning speed."

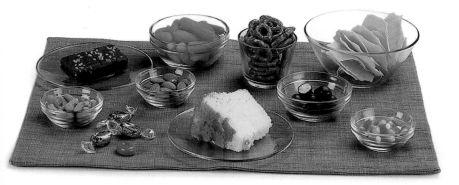

snacks that provide some protein, fiber, or good fat will help turn down your appetite. So when you feel your stomach rumbling, turn to a stick of string cheese, a hard-boiled egg, raw vegetables, or nuts over what's available in the vending machine.

treats

Make sure to enjoy a delicious treat every day! If you stop eating yummy things, you set yourself up for bingeing. And that is not your goal.

You might not find these little goodies in health food stores, but that doesn't mean they can't make a nice addition to your lunch or dinner. Most of my clients save their treat for after dinner.

Consult my Cruise Down Plate food lists on pages 244–45

for optimal treats. I list some of the most highly craved foods from chocolate to ice cream to gingersnaps. As long as you hold yourself to a small serving, you can eat any treat you crave and stay healthy and lose weight. My food lists will suggest the right serving size, so you never have to count calories or consult a nutrition facts label.

To prevent yourself from overdoing it with treats, heed the following tips when you feel a craving coming on.

1. Ask yourself if you really are hungry or if you really are craving emotional comfort and nurturing. If it's emotional, then make sure to activate The People Solution from chapter 3. The true source of most cravings is an emotional craving for nurturing and comfort. So don't worry—

since you have finished chapter 3, you will do great!

2. Wait 10 minutes before indulging. Most cravings only last 10 minutes. After that, they disappear. During those 10 minutes, drink a 16-ounce glass of water with lemon and take a few deep breaths. You might even go for a short walk. Many times, water is what your body really needs. The deep breaths will help melt away any stress that might be driving you to eat.

water: your secret weapon

And now for the final secret to the Cruise Down Plate eating system: water.

When you increase your intake of water, your stomach never gets empty. Consequently, you will not have to eat as much food to feel satisfied. Bottom line: Water is an essential, calorie-free secret to feeling satisfied and happy throughout the day.

Why else is water so critical to your weight loss? Well, remember what I said about vegetables being water-rich foods? A glass of water obviously counts, too. And remember that in order for your lean muscle tissue to burn fat, it needs

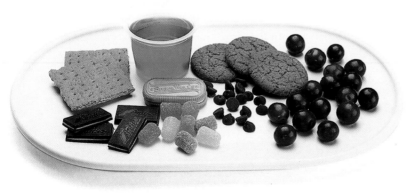

oxygen to help convert the fat into energy. When you drink a glass of water, you will dramatically increase your oxygen levels, improving your metabolism.

And probably the most powerful side effect of drinking

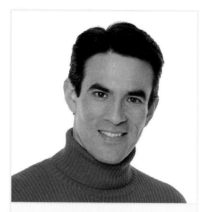

"The Cruise Down Plate will help you to automatically eat the right amount of protein to keep your muscles firm and burning fat."

more water is that your body will operate more efficiently and properly. We all have a series of blood vessels that carry nutrients and oxygen-rich red blood all over our bodies. When you are dehydrated, you start to feel tired because your blood thickens and your heart consequently must work harder to pump blood throughout your body. End result: Oxygen and nutrients don't travel as quickly to your muscles and other organs that need them.

Here's something else. Anytime you feel thirsty, you are already dehydrated. You simply can't rely on your thirst to tell you when to drink a glass of water. That's why I recommend you drink one glass of water each hour throughout your day. When you do this, you will boost your energy level and decrease your appetite.

Though you may have seen recommendations to drink eight 8-ounce glasses of water a day, I suggest you drink much more. Rather than an 8-ounce glass, use a pint glass (16 ounces) and fill it every hour. That is a total of 128 ounces before you leave work and head for home.

That might sound like a lot, but your life will change for the better, and your waistline will soon see the difference. If you

feel you might have to gradually build up to 16 ounces at a time, then start with an 8-ounce glass. Regardless, before you continue to read any more of this book, stand up and drink a tall glass of water right now! I promise you will feel a big difference in just a few minutes.

Stephan and Regina Carey sure did. "Wow! We noticed an immediate difference as soon as we started drinking all this water," they told me. "The water ended up replacing all of the soda we used to drink. Now we've had the same unopened cases of soda in the garage for several months. Water satiates our cravings for food, too. If we are craving something sweet or salty, we drink a big glass of water to wake up our taste buds and figure out what our bodies really need. It makes a huge difference."

Of course, with all this extra water consumption, you will be making some new visits to the bathroom, but that is good. Think of those extra trips to the bathroom as walking time, as your bonus stress reducer and workout for your heart!

simple, easy, and effective

So you see, it is very important that you remember that the only way to make weight loss easier is by not depriving yourself of your favorite foods, not ever going on a starvation diet, and not counting calories.

My challenge for you right now is that you start using your Cruise Down Plate eating system for 28 days and see how great you do. I know you will never go back to your old eating habits. You will be a "Cruiser" for life.

And most important, you will finally step off that dieting roller coaster with its numerous ups and downs. You will never fear food or feel guilty again. You'll eat the foods you love confidently at any restaurant, party, special occasion, or holiday gathering. You will now know how to truly enjoy snacking, including how to snack on chocolate. And most important, with the Cruise Down Plate, you will maximize and ensure your weight loss.

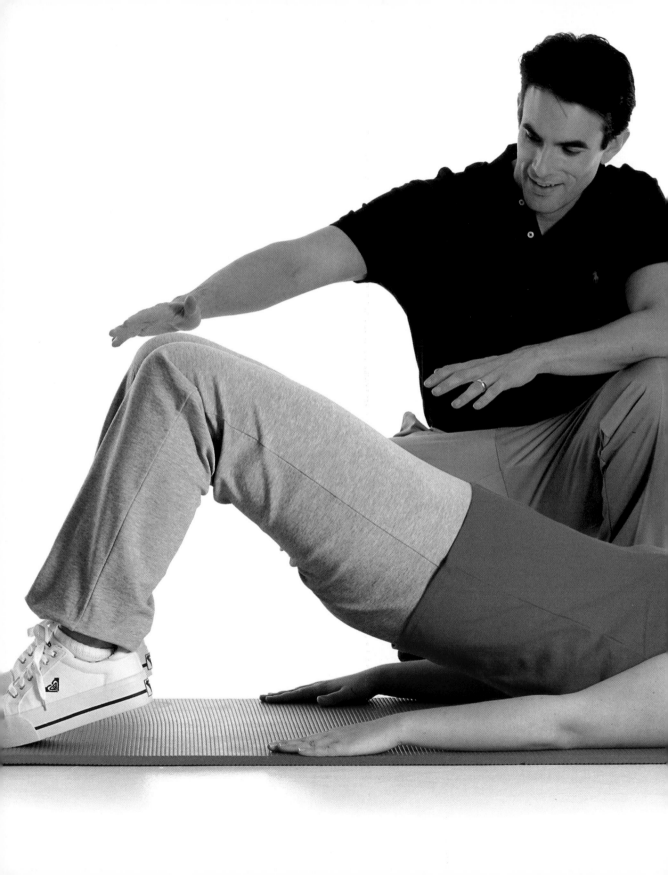

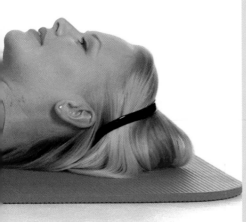

3
The
Program

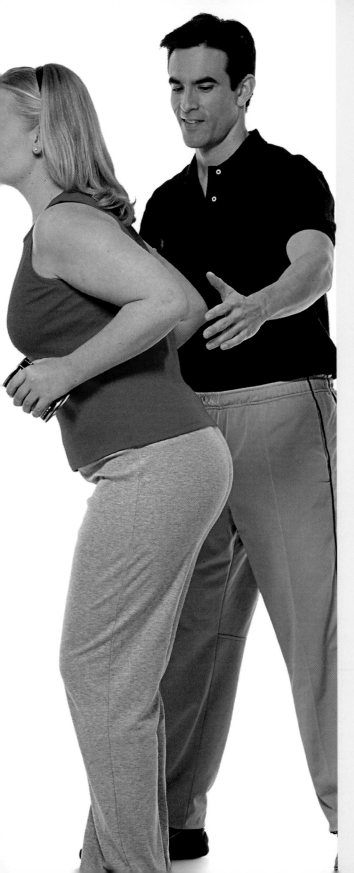

7

4 Weeks to a New You

Putting *8 Minutes in the Morning for Real Shapes, Real Sizes* into Action

your 28-day plan

You're about to tackle the most important part of the *8 Minutes in the Morning for Real Shapes, Real Sizes* program. In this chapter, you and I will meet each day to sculpt your new life and the new you!

your commitment

To succeed in shedding 2 pounds a week, you must follow each day's three steps. Don't skip any aspect of the program. Make that commitment right now. Promise me that you will do that. It's critical for your success.

During the next 28 days, you will learn important secrets that will show you how to better incorporate The People Solution into your life, eliminating emotional eating once and for all. Each day you'll also find two suggested Cruise Moves to do for 8 minutes, and you will also receive

---

critical secrets

week 1: Nurture yourself

week 2: Improve your communication

week 3: Expand your buddy team

week 4: Enjoy your weight-loss adventure

---

a tip to using the Cruise Down Plate. This three-step approach will help you to stay focused and motivated during each day of your journey to a new you.

3 daily steps to success

Each day focuses on three simple steps:

1. Before the 8 minutes: The People Solution

2. The 8 minutes: Cruise Moves

3. After the 8 minutes: The Cruise Down Plate

Let's start with The People Solution, the first step you will take each morning. My daily People Solution tasks will take you just a few minutes to read and complete but will help to powerfully reaffirm and put into action everything you learned in chapter 3. These daily tips will show you how to better support

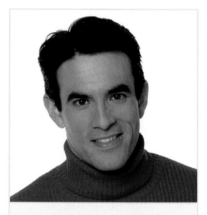

"Never give up, surrender, or quit."

and nurture yourself as well as how to get your inner team to better support you.

Each week, your People Solution tasks focus on a particular theme. During week one, you'll focus on using the power of visualization to better nurture yourself each morning. Week two is all about improving your communication within your inner team. During week three, you will learn secrets to help you further expand your buddy team. And the last week is dedicated to great resources and tools to make your weight-loss adventure more enjoyable. To hear me personally talk you through any of these visualizations, visit www.jorgecruise.com.

Your second step each morning will be your Cruise Moves. These take just 8 minutes. Before your Cruise Moves, warm up by jogging or marching in place for a minute or two. When doing the Cruise Moves, always remember to never lock your joints. Always keep them soft. Breathe normally, and make sure your shoulders are relaxed (not hunched toward your ears), your abdominals are firm, and

your spine is long and extended. You can always use a towel or exercise mat when you're on the floor. Then, after your Cruise Moves, cool down with the stretches suggested below.

During your final step each morning, you'll learn how to make your Cruise Down Plate eating routine even more delicious and simple.

Ideally, start the program on a Monday. That will allow you to take every Sunday off from your Cruise Moves (but not from your People Solution or Cruise Down Plate), giving you an opportunity to rest, weigh in, and prepare for

the next week. Before starting on your 28-day journey, make sure you have done the following:

• Photocopied 28 days' worth of the master Cruise Weight-Loss Planner on page 246.

• Found comfortable clothing to wear for your Cruise Moves (your PJs are perfect).

• Taken your "before" and "after" photos and taped them onto pages 46–47.

• Calculated your goal weight and goal date and written them on page 45.

Ready? Let's get started!

YOUR COOLDOWN

After your Cruise Moves, do the following stretches to cool down and increase your flexibility.

Sky-reaching pose: Stand tall and reach with both hands toward the sky as high as you comfortably can. Feel the stretch lengthening your spine, bringing more range of motion to your joints. Breathe deeply through your nose. Hold from 10 seconds to 1 minute.

Cobra stretch: Lie on a mat on your belly with your palms flat on the ground next to your shoulders and your legs just slightly less than shoulder-width apart. Lift your upper body up off the ground, inhaling through your nose as

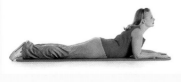

you rise. Press your hips into the floor and curve your upper body backward, looking up. Again, do the best you can. Hold from 10 seconds to 1 minute.

Hurdler's stretch: Sit on a mat on the floor with your legs extended in front of you. Keeping your back straight, gently bend forward from the hips and reach as far as you can toward your toes. If possible, pull your toes back slightly toward your upper body. Do the best you can—don't worry if this stretch is difficult for you right now. Eventually, you'll get it! Hold from 10 seconds to 1 minute.

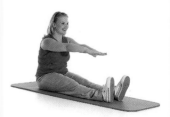

WEEK1
day1

"*A man is what he thinks about all day long.*"

Ralph Waldo Emerson

the people solution

For the next 7 days, you and I will focus on nurturing your inner motivation by using powerful visualization techniques. Visualization helps you see yourself in the future—in this case, after you've reached your goal weight. Each time you see your future success, you steal a bit of that powerful positive energy and experience it today. It's magical.

your best birthday

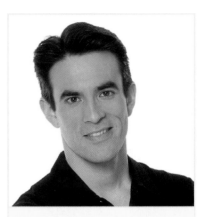

Let's take a look at a birthday in the future after you've reached your goal weight. Do the following with me for just a few minutes:

• Close your eyes and take a few deep, relaxing breaths—in through your nose and out through your mouth. Smile because we are about to jump into the future!

• With your eyes closed, imagine that today is your birthday, the first birthday you are celebrating after reaching your goal weight. Imagine you have just arrived at big surprise party. Imagine your birthday as a film in color. More than 50 people fill the room. You feel great and look fantastic. You're wearing a great outfit that you bought earlier that day. What are people saying to you? Hear the compliments they're telling you about how healthy and vibrant you look? How big is your smile right now?

> "Each time you see your future success, you steal a bit of that powerful positive energy and experience it today."

cruise moves
chest and back

a: squeeze hold

Sit in a sturdy chair (one without wheels) with your feet flat on the floor. Bend your arms and exhale as you press the palms of your hands together at chest level. Once in position, keep your chest tight and flexed. Hold firmly for up to 60 seconds as you breathe normally.

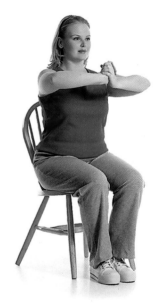

the cruise down plate: chew your food

Here's a great Cruise Down Plate trick: Chew each bite of your meal between 20 and 30 times before swallowing. Count in your head while you're chewing until you become conditioned to do it naturally.

Chewing your food for a longer period of time aids digestion by stimulating your salivary glands to break down the food even more. It also will prevent overeating because you must spend more time on each bite. The more slowly you eat, the faster you will feel full and satiated. (Remember all those hormones, like leptin and cholecystokinin?) This trick might not make you a great dinner conversationalist, but your body will thank you for it!

Hurdler's stretch

Cobra stretch

b:

Sit 2

chair

forwa

palms

press

to 60 second

★ **THE MIRACLE PRAYER** ★

Lord Jesus, I come before you, just as I am. I am sorry for
sins, I repent of my sins, please forgive me. In your name,
orgive all others for what they have done against me. I
ounce satan, the evil spirits and all their works. I give you
entire self. Lord Jesus, now and forever, I invite you into
life Jesus, I accept you as my Lord, God and Saviour. Heal
change me, strengthen me in body, soul and spirit.
Come Lord Jesus, cover me with your precious blood, and
me with your **Holy Spirit, I Love You Lord Jesus. I**
ise You Jesus. I Thank You Jesus.** I shall follow you
ry day of my life. Amen.

Mary my mother, Queen of Peace, St. Peregrine, the cancer
t, all you Angels and Saints please help me. Amen.

primatur † Francisco Maria Aguilera Gonzalez, Auxiliary
Bishop of Mexico, September 8, 1992

this Prayer faithfully, no matter how you feel, when you
e to the point where you sincerely mean each word, with
your heart, something good spiritually will happen to you.
will experience Jesus, and HE will change your whole
in a very special way. You will see.

© 1993 Servite Fathers, O.S.M.

With prayers, thanks and love
Fr. Peter Mary Rookey, O.S.M.,
International Compassion Ministry
20180 Governors Hwy., Room 203
Olympia Fields, Illinois 60461-1067
(708) 748-MARY (6279)

today's journa

WEEK1
day2

> "I believe that when you realize who you really are, you understand that nothing can stop you from becoming that person."
>
> **Christine Lincoln**

the people solution

Are you ready for another night of partying and celebration? Are you ready to let your hair down and party like you have never done before? Well, you are about to be invited to the most exciting New Year's Eve celebration in your life!

celebrate new year's eve

Let's take a look at a future New Year's Eve, after you've reached your goal weight. Do the following with me for just a few minutes:

• Close your eyes and take a few deep, relaxing breaths—in through your nose and out through your mouth. Smile because we are about to jump into the future!

• Imagine that today is December 31. This is the first New Year's Eve that you celebrate the new you at your new weight. See yourself at your favorite shopping mall. What dress or outfit will you buy? How long have you been looking forward to buying this new dress or outfit? What does it look like?

• Jump a few more hours into the future and see yourself at a grand, Cinderella-type ball. What band is playing? What songs are they singing? See your best friends and family there with you. See the huge smiles on their faces when they see how absolutely wonderful you look. Hear the compliments they share with you. Hear them tell you, "I am so proud of you." See your sparkling smile.

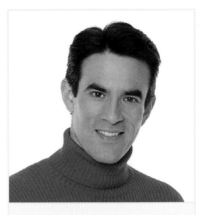

"This program is all about being healthy, not about being superskinny."

cruise moves
shoulders and
abdominals

8-MINUTE LOG				
exercise	set 1	set 2	set 3	set 4
a				
b				

a: glide hold

You can do this move while sitting or standing. Exhale and raise your arms out to your sides. Stop once your hands reach shoulder height. Hold firmly for up to 60 seconds, breathing normally. Try to keep your shoulders relaxed away from your ears. This move may look simple, but you will feel the burn.

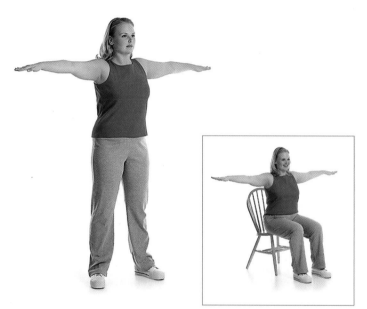

the cruise down plate: the best condiment

People often ask me what condiment to use in place of mayonnaise and other high-fat dips and spreads. I answer, "Salsa." Not just for tortilla chips anymore, salsa provides a terrific topping for your vegetables, proteins, and anything else that needs a little kick of flavor. Salsa adds a wallop of flavor, but only a minimal number of calories, to your food. In fact, a tablespoon of low-fat salsa has only 5 calories!

exercise sequence

warm up

Jog or march in place.

cruise moves

Do one 60-second repetition of Cruise Move (a), then immediately

do one 60-second repetition of Cruise Move (b). Repeat this cycle 4 times, and you will be done in 8 minutes.

cool down

After your Cruise Moves, do these stretches (see page 107).

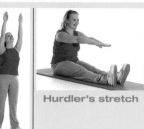

Sky-reaching pose

Hurdler's stretch

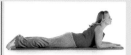

Cobra stretch

b: stir hold

Sit or stand with good posture. Lengthen your spine and straighten your back. Relax your shoulders. Exhale as you tighten your abdominal muscles. Make a fist with one of your hands and rub the bottom part of your fist in a circle over the center of your belly button area (as if you were stirring cake batter). This will force you to keep your abs contracted strongly. Hold for up to 60 seconds, breathing normally.

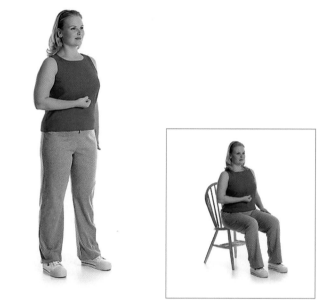

today's journal

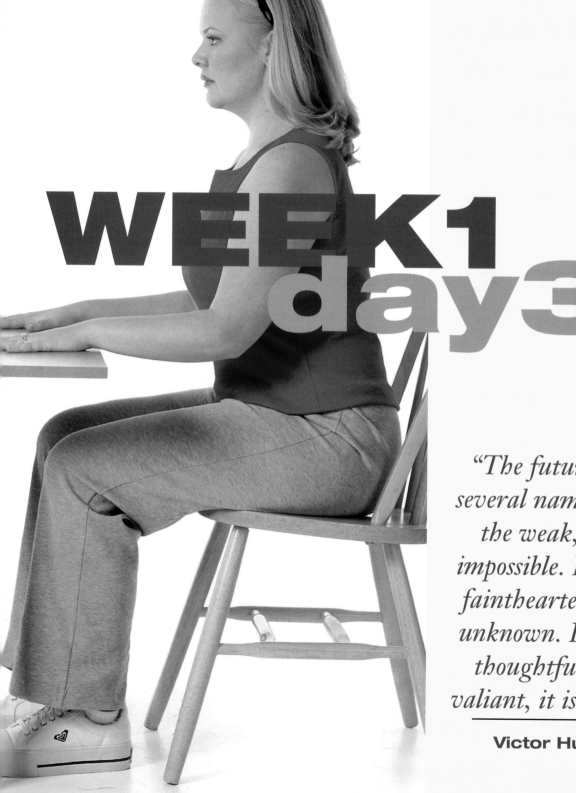

WEEK1
day3

"The future has several names. For the weak, it is impossible. For the fainthearted, it is unknown. For the thoughtful and valiant, it is ideal."

Victor Hugo

the people solution

It's time for you to take the vacation of your lifetime! Get ready to go to the place you have always wanted to visit. You will travel first-class with your family and best friends, or perhaps just by yourself.

the vacation of your lifetime

Let's take a look at a future dream vacation, after you've reached your goal weight. Do the following with me for just a few minutes:

• Close your eyes and take a few deep, relaxing breaths—in through your nose and out through your mouth.

• Imagine you have just arrived at your dream vacation spot. Are you at a beach in the Caribbean or in Hawaii? How blue is the water? How warm is the sand under your feet? Or are you in Paris atop the Eiffel Tower? How magnificent is the view?

There are no limits to what you can do. You can stroll or run or dance or walk anywhere and talk to and meet anyone. Perhaps you meet a new best friend, someone you have been waiting to meet your entire life. How big is your smile right now?

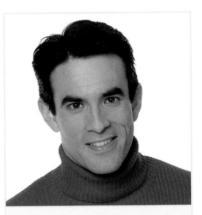

"There are no limits to what you can do."

cruise moves
triceps and biceps

8-MINUTE LOG				
exercise	set 1	set 2	set 3	set 4
a				
b				

a: push-down hold

Sit about 2 feet in front of a table in a sturdy chair (one without wheels) with your feet flat on the floor. Place your palms on the table with your elbows bent about 90 degrees. Exhale as you press down into the tabletop as hard as you can. Hold for up to 60 seconds, breathing normally.

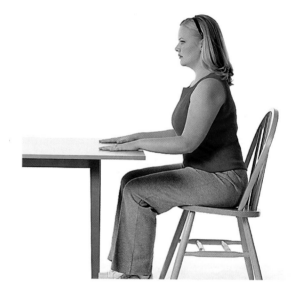

the cruise down plate: coffee shop caution

Your local coffee shop is a huge fat trap. Most coffee drinks are higher in calories than cheeseburgers! An average tall cappuccino is packed with 140 calories and 7 grams of fat. Worse, a venti mocha contains 510 calories and 27 grams of fat! These drinks are blended with chocolate, full-fat milk, whipped cream, and sugary syrups. So stay away from this hidden fat trap and stick with tea or plain coffee.

exercise sequence

warm up

Jog or march in place.

cruise moves

Do one 60-second repetition of Cruise Move (a), then immediately

do one 60-second repetition of Cruise Move (b). Repeat this cycle 4 times, and you will be done in 8 minutes.

cool down

After your Cruise Moves, do these stretches (see page 107).

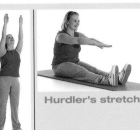

Sky-reaching pose

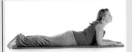

Hurdler's stretch

Cobra stretch

b: lift hold

While still seated in front of the table, place your palms under the tabletop with your elbows bent about 90 degrees. Push up on the underside of the table as hard as you can. Hold for up to 60 seconds as you breathe normally.

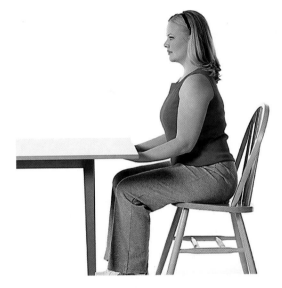

today's journal

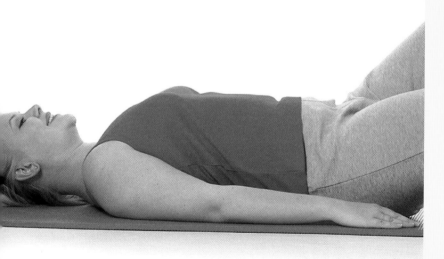

WEEK1
day4

> "Never fear the space between your dreams and reality. If you can dream it, you can make it so."

Belva Davis

the people solution

After your perfect vacation, it's time to come home. You're now at the airport, and you are about to bump in to an old friend, maybe a high school classmate or old boyfriend or girlfriend whom you have not seen in years. This person has not yet seen the new you!

surprise an old friend

Do the following with me for just a few minutes:

• Close your eyes and take a few relaxing breaths—in through your nose and out through your mouth. Smile because we are about to jump into the future!

• Imagine you are coming home from your extraordinary vacation. You look rested, healthy, and happier than ever. As you

board your plane, you bump into someone. When this person sees you, his or her eyes open wide. This person has not seen you since you have lost the weight. Hear your old friend say, "Oh my gosh, you look amazing! What did you do?" Your friend looks and sounds stunned by how incredible you look. How big is your smile right now?

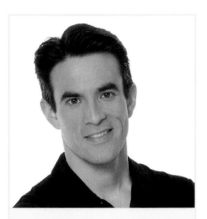

"Your [long-lost] friend looks and sounds stunned by how incredible you look."

cruise moves
hamstrings and quadriceps

8-MINUTE LOG				
exercise	set 1	set 2	set 3	set 4
a				
b				

a: long bridge hold

Lie with your back on an exercise mat or towel. Rest your arms at your sides and extend your legs. Bend your knees slightly. Press into your heels as you exhale and lift your hips about 2 inches from the floor. Imagine you are a long bridge, like the Golden Gate Bridge in San Francisco. Hold for up to 60 seconds as you breathe normally.

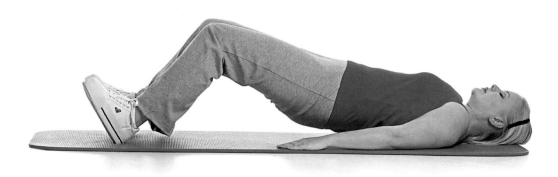

the cruise down plate: frozen veggies

Always keep your freezer stocked with frozen vegetables. Frozen veggies are a convenient and cost-effective alternative to fresh veggies, and they're still packed with all the fiber and nutrients you need. Most frozen veggies don't need to be washed and are already chopped into ready-to-eat pieces. Toss frozen veggies into your soups, stir-fries, pasta sauces, or anything else that you'll be simmering on the stove.

exercise sequence

warm up

Jog or march in place.

cruise moves

Do one 60-second repetition of Cruise Move (a), then immediately

do one 60-second repetition of Cruise Move (b). Repeat this cycle 4 times, and you will be done in 8 minutes.

cool down

After your Cruise Moves, do these stretches (see page 107).

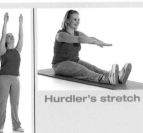

Sky-reaching pose

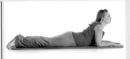

Hurdler's stretch

Cobra stretch

b: one leg hold

While still lying on your back, bend your knees and place your feet flat on the floor. Lift and extend your left leg about 1 foot from the floor. Hold for 30 to 60 seconds as you breathe normally. You should feel it burn on the upper part of your leg. Lower your leg and repeat with your right leg.

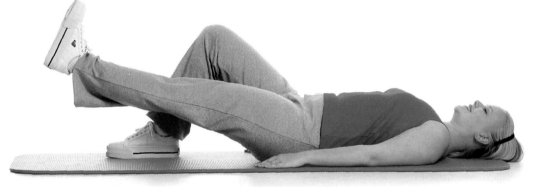

today's journal

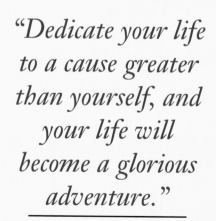

WEEK1
day5

"Dedicate your life to a cause greater than yourself, and your life will become a glorious adventure."

Mack Douglas

the people solution

Today will be one of the proudest and most gratifying days of your life. You are about to see the tears of joys in the eyes of someone *you* have helped to lose weight. You took this person under your wing after you reached your goal weight. Now you have helped this friend change his or her life.

touch a life,
become a role model

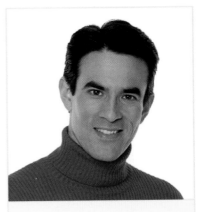

Do the following with me for just a few minutes:

• Close your eyes and take a few deep, relaxing breaths—in through your nose and out through your mouth. Smile because we are about to jump into the future!

• Imagine your friend has invited you to dinner to thank you for helping him or her to lose more than 30 pounds. Before you know it, your friend raises his or her glass in the air and makes a toast, a toast that causes both of you to break down in tears. Your friend says, "To my best friend, a friend who has supported me and comforted me when things where difficult. To a friend who has helped me flourish. Thank you . . . thank you . . . thank you."

• See your tears of joy. Feel them run down your cheek. How proud are you at this moment?

"Today will be one of the proudest and most gratifying days of your life."

cruise moves
calves and butt

8-MINUTE LOG				
exercise	set 1	set 2	set 3	set 4
a				
b				

a: high-heel hold

Stand with your feet directly under your hips. Exhale as you lift your heels, rising onto the balls of your feet. Pretend you are wearing very high heels. (Place one hand on a sturdy chair or wall for balance.) Hold for 60 seconds.

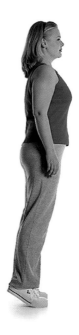

the cruise down plate: a slimming cereal winner

I love cereals with whole grains and minimal processing. My favorite is called Uncle Sam Cereal. I love it because it contains both whole-grain wheat and flax seeds. Whole grains have a low glycemic index, which helps support weight loss. The flax seeds, which contain omega-3 fatty acids, help curb appetite. (Return to chapter 6 to read more about the benefits of flax.) Uncle Sam Cereal was awarded the Seal of Approval from the Glycemic Research In- stitute in Washington, D.C., as a food that does not overly stimulate blood glucose and insulin and does not stimulate fat-storing enzymes. Find out more about this great cereal at www.jorgecruise.com/unclesam.

exercise sequence

warm up

Jog or march in place.

cruise moves

Do one 60-second repetition of Cruise Move (a), then immediately

do one 60-second repetition of Cruise Move (b). Repeat this cycle 4 times, and you will be done in 8 minutes.

cool down

After your Cruise Moves, do these stretches (see page 107).

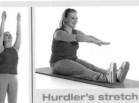

Sky-reaching pose

Hurdler's stretch

Cobra stretch

b: standing butt squeeze hold

Stand with your feet directly under your hips and your arms resting at your sides. Check your posture. Make sure your back is long and straight, your abdominals are firm, and your shoulders are relaxed away from your ears. Squeeze your buttocks muscles as tight as you can. Hold for 60 seconds. Though this move seems extremely simple, it really works!

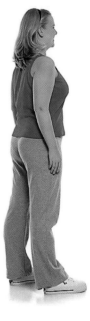

today's journal

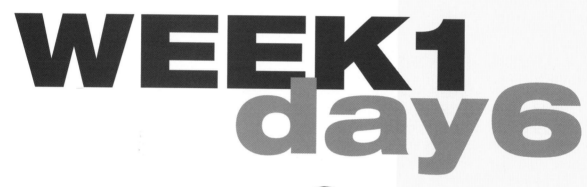

WEEK1
day6

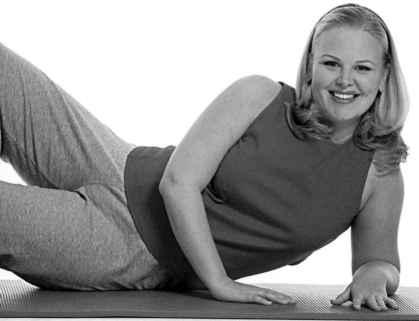

"We've got two lives. The one we're given and the one we make."

Kobi Yamada

the people solution

Today is the day you will be personally recognized by me! Each year I host a red rose ceremony in San Diego for my most successful clients. My staff and I pick only 20 people to fly to San Diego, where I meet with them and hear their weight-loss stories. The red rose ceremony takes place in front of 200 other people who want to lose weight. My camera crew films this happy event so that I can share it with people all over America on my television appearances. Are you ready to join me on stage?

become a tv star!

Do the following with me for just a few minutes:

• Close your eyes and take a few deep, relaxing breaths—in through your nose and out through your mouth.

• Imagine you are visiting San Diego. You are in a large auditorium with hundreds of other people. You look stunning, and you and I are about to meet. I call your name as I hold your red rose and your "before" and "after" photos. I share with the group how many pounds you have lost. The crowd cheers! I say, "Come on up." As you walk on to the stage the crowd cheers even louder. You and I meet, and I give you your rose. How big is your smile right now?

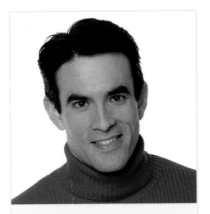

"To find out more about the red rose ceremony, turn to page 247."

cruise moves
inner and outer thighs

8-MINUTE LOG				
exercise	set 1	set 2	set 3	set 4
a				
b				

a: inner-rise hold

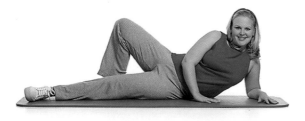
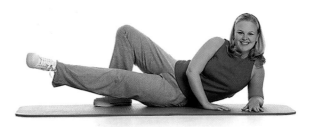

1 Lie on an exercise mat on your left side with your legs extended. Support your body weight on your left forearm. Rest your right hand on the mat in front of your tummy for support.

2 Bend your right knee and place your right foot on the mat behind your left leg. Lift your extended left leg about 1 foot off the mat. Hold for 30 to 60 seconds, breathing normally. Then switch sides and repeat with your other leg.

the cruise down plate: eat with chopsticks

Push that fork aside and grab some chopsticks. No, I'm not talking about filling your plate with chow mein and moo shoo pork. Rather, use your chopsticks to eat *all* foods.

Chopsticks force you to eat smaller bites at a slower pace. Since chopsticks cannot pick up as much food as a fork, you must put less food in your mouth at a time, which makes you chew

more often. You'll find yourself fuller and more satisfied with less food.

exercise sequence

warm up

Jog or march in place.

cruise moves

Do one 60-second repetition of Cruise Move (a), then immediately

do one 60-second repetition of Cruise Move (b). Repeat this cycle 4 times, and you will be done in 8 minutes.

cool down

After your Cruise Moves, do these stretches (see page 107).

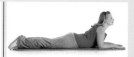

Sky-reaching pose

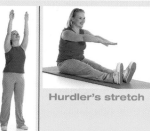

Hurdler's stretch

Cobra stretch

b: outer-rise hold

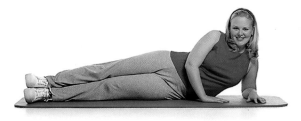

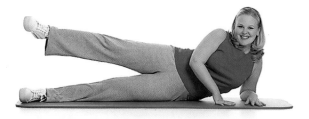

1 While still lying on the mat on your left side with your legs extended, support your body weight on your left forearm. Rest your right hand on the mat in front of your tummy for support.

2 Lift your extended right leg about 1 foot above your left leg. Hold for 30 to 60 seconds, breathing normally. Lower and then switch sides and repeat by lifting your other leg.

today's journal

WEEK 1 day 7

"Starting each day I shall try to learn something new about me and about you and about the world I live in, so that I may continue to experience all things as if they have been newly born."

Leo Buscaglia

the people solution

It's time to record your first week's progress. This will help to keep you focused and motivated. If you'd like to share your progress with me, send an e-mail with your answers to firstweek@jorgecruise.com.

capture your progress

Grab a pen and answer the following questions. Then share this with your accountability buddy. If you need more space, turn the page and continue writing in Today's Journal.

1. What is your current weight?
_____

2. What was your original weight?
_____

3. What have you done well this week? What makes you proud of you?
_____
_____
_____
_____
_____
_____

4. What could you improve next week?
_____
_____
_____
_____
_____
_____
_____

5. What is your game plan for week 2?
_____
_____
_____
_____
_____
_____
_____

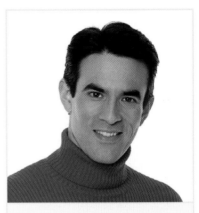

"I will e-mail you tips on how to make week 2 even more fun and effective."

cruise moves
your day off

I just found my New Year's goals from last year. For the past several years I have tried to lose 10 pounds as one of my goals. But it never happened. This year I tripled the 10 pounds—losing 30 pounds in all. It feels great!

"I even won a weight-loss bet with my brother and won $100!"

I am a single parent, go to school full-time, and work part-time. Jorge's program really fits into my busy lifestyle. It really works!

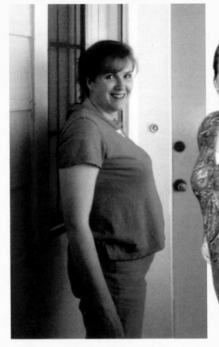

Elyse lost the weight and won a bet.

the cruise down plate

One slice of watermelon is a sweet pick for your morning Cruise Down Plate fruit serving. Because it contains so much water, watermelon is low in calories. One cup has only 50 calories!

prevent cancer with watermelon

Watermelon is also packed with disease-fighting vitamins such as A, B6, and C, along with magnesium, folate, and potassium—all important heart disease and cancer fighters. Folate also prevents birth defects. Finally, watermelon contains lots of lycopene, an important plant chemical that can lower your risk of certain cancers and help fight heart disease.

To choose the best watermelon, buy it whole rather than presliced. As the inside of the melon is exposed to light, the healthful nutrients break down. Look for watermelon with an asymmetrical shape. The melon should be firm to the touch, without any bruises, cuts, or soft spots. Pick up the melon to check its weight. It should feel fairly heavy for its size. Turn it over to check for a lighter yellow spot on the melon's underside. This marks the spot where the melon sat on the ground and ripened in the sun for you to enjoy. Once you cut up the melon, cover it and refrigerate it to prevent the nutrients from breaking down.

today's journal

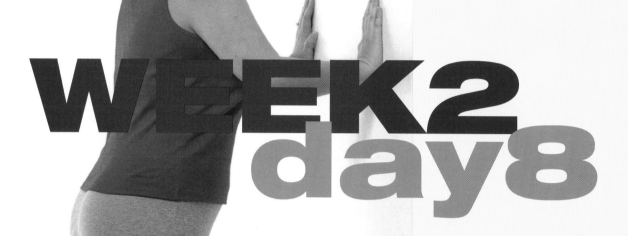

WEEK2
day8

> "To lose one's health renders science null, art inglorious, strength unavailing, wealth useless, and eloquence powerless."

Herophilus, c. 300 B.C.

the people solution

Have you already mailed copies of your Power Pledge Poster, your healthy weight goal dates, and your Day in the Life of the Future Me essay to your e-mail buddies, phone buddies, and accountability buddy? If you haven't, do that right now.

the power of "thank you"

In order for them to best support you, your buddies must have those items. You cannot complete the following exercise until you have first mailed those materials because today, you will send a thank-you note to your seven buddies. You cannot believe how happy your inner team will feel once they see you have taken the extra time to mail a handwritten note (not an e-mail).

Your thank-you note does not have to be fancy. Write your note on stationery, a specific "thank-you" card from a card store, or on regular notebook paper. Tell your buddies specific details about how they have helped you during the past 7 days. Thank them for their time, effort, and support. Make this your first of many thank-you notes. That is one of the most simple and powerful secrets to maintaining good friends.

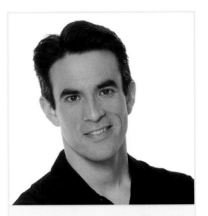

"Say 'thank you' often, and your buddies will become your most cherished supporters."

cruise moves
chest and back

a: wall pump

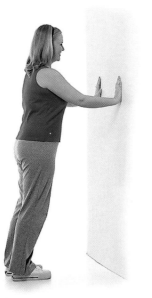

1 Stand at arms' length away from a wall with your feet directly under your hips. Lean forward and place your palms against the wall. Your elbows should be slightly bent.

2 Inhale as you slowly bend your elbows, bringing your chest and torso closer to the wall. Exhale as you slowly press yourself back to the starting position, straightening your arms as you go. Slowly repeat for 60 seconds.

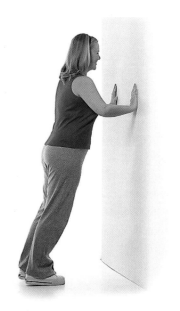

the cruise down plate: the magic of a tiny bag

Green tea is brewed from the same leaves as black tea. Green tea, however, is made by steaming and drying the leaves right after picking rather than fermenting them first. Tea is good for both your heart and your waistline. Though all types of tea contain antioxidants that protect your heart and slightly boost your metabolism, green tea may be the healthiest.

Studies have shown that green tea can boost how many calories you burn by up to 4 percent in a 24-hour period. Over the course of a year, that can add up to an extra pound or two of burned fat. (Be aware that green tea does contain caffeine, though it's less than half the amount of coffee.)

exercise sequence

warm up

Jog or march in place.

cruise moves

Do one 60-second repetition of Cruise Move (a), then immediately

do one 60-second repetition of Cruise Move (b). Repeat this cycle 4 times, and you will be done in 8 minutes.

cool down

After your Cruise Moves, do these stretches (see page 107).

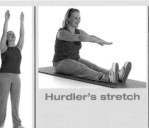

Sky-reaching pose

Hurdler's stretch

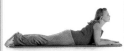

Cobra stretch

b: superman hold

Stand in front of a sturdy chair. Your right foot should be directly under your right hip. Now bend forward and place your right palm on the chair's seat, just under your right shoulder. Exhale as you raise and extend your left leg back and your left arm forward, forming a straight line from foot to fingertips. Hold for 30 to 60 seconds, then repeat on the other side.

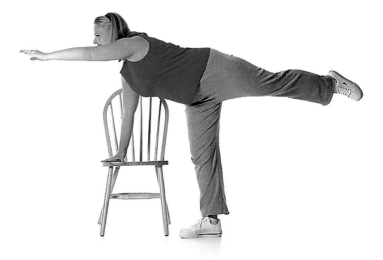

today's journal

WEEK2
day9

> *"If you accept your limitations, you never go beyond them."*
>
> **Brendan Francis**

the people solution

I have a good friend who once worked at Disneyland at a concession stand. Although it wasn't the highest paying job, she loved it more than any other job because everywhere else, she was just an employee. At the park, however, she was a *cast member*. She gave herself the nickname of a performer, and it changed her entire focus at work.

use a nickname

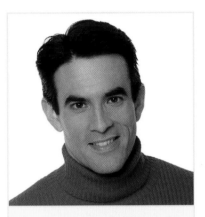

For you to achieve your ideal body, you too must create a positive nickname for yourself, a nickname that gets you excited about exercising and eating well. Too many people unconsciously label themselves in ways that make them feel bad: over the hill, overeater, couch potato, and so on.

I want you to select a positive nickname for yourself. Make up something that works for you. Then, ask your buddy team to call you by this nickname. Every time they refer to you by your new nickname, it will help to fuel your motivation and your success!

"Choose a nickname for yourself. Post it everywhere and ask your buddies to call you by this name."

nicknames

Here are a few examples to get you started:

Sexy Mama

Adonis

Hot Babe

Strong Power Mom

Superwoman

Stud

Your choice _____

cruise moves
shoulders and
abdominals

8-MINUTE LOG				
exercise	set 1	set 2	set 3	set 4
a				
b				

a: bird pump

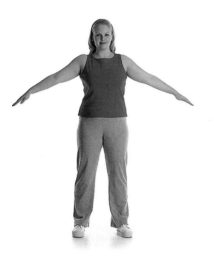

1 Stand with your feet directly under your hips and your arms resting at your sides. Raise and extend your arms about 45 degrees out from your hips. Make sure your shoulders are relaxed, your tummy is firm, and your upper back is straight.

2 Exhale as you raise your arms about 45 degrees above shoulder level. Inhale as you lower them to the starting position. Slowly repeat for 60 seconds.

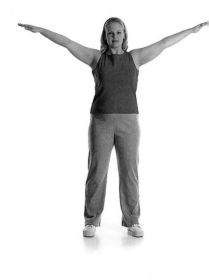

the cruise down plate: drink more water

I just can't say enough about how crucial it is to drink your water every day.

To encourage yourself to drink more water each day, make sure you like the taste of the water you're trying. Sometimes tap water leaves a chemical or mineral aftertaste. In that case, switch to bottled water. People often ask me what brand of bottled water I use. I answer: "Penta." It is ultrapurified water. You see, a lot of bottled waters call themselves "natural," but Penta uses a special process that purifies water without chemicals or additives. And Penta is free of the hundreds of chemicals that may be found in your tap water! For your cells to get their optimal hydration, only the purest water is the way to go.

exercise sequence

warm up

Jog or march in place.

cruise moves

Do one 60-second repetition of Cruise Move (a), then immediately

do one 60-second repetition of Cruise Move (b). Repeat this cycle 4 times, and you will be done in 8 minutes.

cool down

After your Cruise Moves, do these stretches (see page 107).

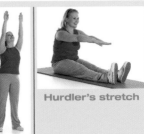

Sky-reaching pose

Hurdler's stretch

Cobra stretch

b: belly breath pump

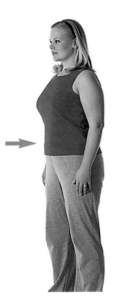

1 Stand with your feet directly under your hips. As you exhale, contract and press your tummy muscles inward as you slowly squeeze all the breath out of your lungs.

2 Reverse the motion by relaxing your tummy outward to slowly pull air into your lungs. Repeat for 60 seconds, breathing slowly, fully emptying and filling your lungs with the effort of your abdominals.

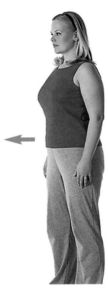

today's journal

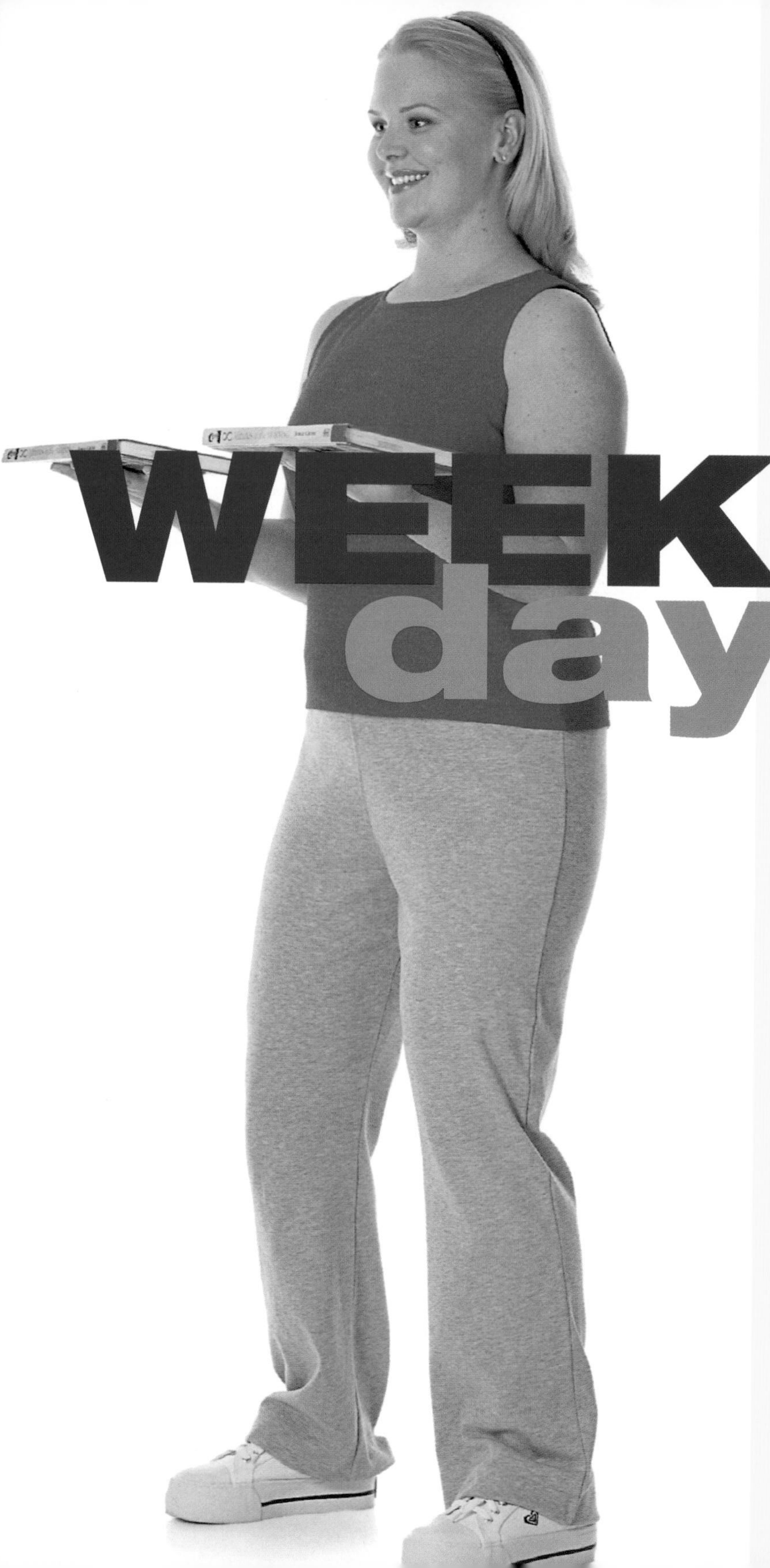

WEEK2
day10

"We are each
responsible for
our own life—
no other person
is or even can be."

Oprah Winfrey

the people solution

Certain words will give you an edge in communicating with your inner team, whereas other words break down your ability to communicate. There are four words that you need to avoid and four words you need to maximize in order to be a successful communicator with your inner team, as well as yourself.

the vocabulary of success

To communicate effectively, avoid saying that you *should* do something or that you *can't* do something or that you will *try* to do something or that you *hope* you can do something. That is not the language of a winner.

Rather, stand tall when communicating with your inner team and yourself. Tell yourself and your inner team that you *will* make it happen, that you *must* make it happen, that you *can* make it happen, and that you *know* you will lose the weight.

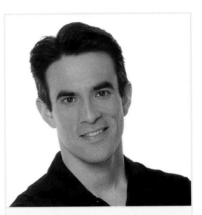

"Use positive words when communicating with your inner team, and you will change your life."

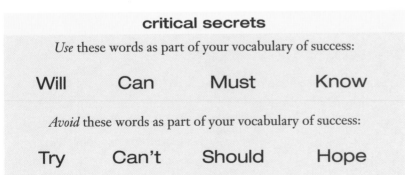

critical secrets

Use these words as part of your vocabulary of success:

Will	Can	Must	Know

Avoid these words as part of your vocabulary of success:

Try	Can't	Should	Hope

cruise moves
triceps and biceps

a: kickback hold

Stand with your feet directly under your hips. Bend forward from your hips about 45 degrees with your arms extended behind you, toward the floor. Exhale as you lift your extended arms behind your torso. Stop once you've extended your arms, but before you've locked your elbows. Hold for 60 seconds.

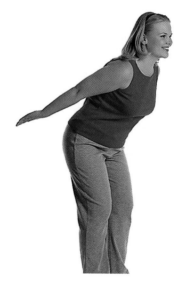

the cruise down plate: fish secrets

If you've never bought and cooked fish before, give it a try. Buy an easy starter fish such as salmon, swordfish, or tuna. These all come in steaks, so they're easy to grill. When buying fish, look for cuts that are moist and firm, with no dried-out edges. If it has skin, it should be shiny and metallic-looking. And it should never smell fishy.

When you get the fish home, marinate it in a combination of miso paste (a soy product), balsamic vinegar, olive oil, and a touch of soy sauce for 45 minutes and pop it on the grill. Enjoy!

exercise sequence

warm up

Jog or march in place.

cruise moves

Do one 60-second repetition of Cruise Move (a), then immediately

do one 60-second repetition of Cruise Move (b). Repeat this cycle 4 times, and you will be done in 8 minutes.

cool down

After your Cruise Moves, do these stretches (see page 107).

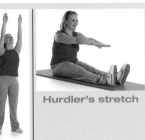

Sky-reaching pose

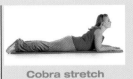

Hurdler's stretch

Cobra stretch

b: book hold

Stand with your feet directly under your hips. Balance a heavy textbook or phone book in each hand with your palms facing up and your arms bent at 90 degrees. Hold for up to 60 seconds as you breathe normally, keeping your back long and straight and your abdominals firm.

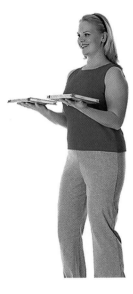

today's journal _____

WEEK2
day11

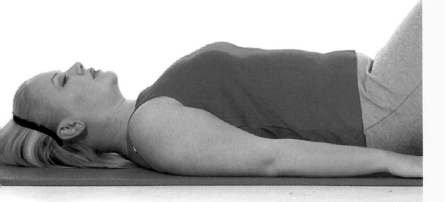

"Diseases can be our spiritual flat tires disruptions in our lives that seem to be disasters at the time but end by redirecting our lives in a meaningful way."

Bernie Siegel, M.D.

the people solution

Symbols carry a lot of power. For example, what has more power, the word "Christian" or a cross; the word "Jew" or the Star of David?

the power of metaphors

Some language symbols, called metaphors, are so powerful that they can help or hurt your communication with your inner team, depending on which language symbols you use.

The number one metaphor that I hear from my new clients is, "I have to win this *battle* with weight." How joyful and happy are you when you think of battles? Battles are hard and difficult. That is not my idea of a positive frame of mind.

But what would happen if you turned the battle into a game?

Or, better yet, into an adventure? What if every time you talked with your inner team this week you referred to your weight loss as an adventure? Your attitude and perspective would certainly improve. Still not sure if changing this one metaphor will change your life? Well, tonight go out and rent the Academy Award–winning Italian movie *Life Is Beautiful*. Once you see the movie, you will fully realize the power of looking at life in a positive light.

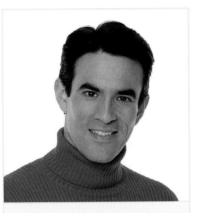

"Every time you talk with your inner team this week, refer to your weight loss as an adventure."

cruise moves
hamstrings and
quadriceps

a: leg lift pump

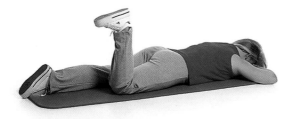 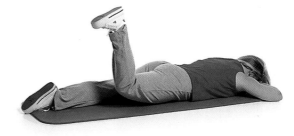

1 Lie on your tummy with your legs extended and arms bent comfortably. Rest your forehead on your wrists or forearms. Bend your right leg 90 degrees, so that the bottom of your right foot faces the ceiling and your right thigh remains in contact with your mat.

2 Exhale as you press your right foot up. You might not be able to lift it very far, but you'll really work the back of your thigh and butt in the process. Inhale as you lower, repeat for 30 to 60 seconds. Now switch legs.

the cruise down plate: chew gum while you cook

Many of us can't stand to be in the kitchen without nibbling, tasting, or testing what's being prepared. By the time dinner is ready, you might have unknowingly already consumed half your meal's worth of calories while standing at the stove! By popping a stick of sugarless gum into your mouth while you cook, you'll keep your mouth busy and prevent yourself from nibbling. So chew gum while you cook and save your meal for your plate.

exercise sequence

warm up

Jog or march in place.

cruise moves

Do one 60-second repetition of Cruise Move (a), then immediately

do one 60-second repetition of Cruise Move (b). Repeat this cycle 4 times, and you will be done in 8 minutes.

cool down

After your Cruise Moves, do these stretches (see page 107).

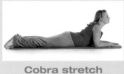

Sky-reaching pose

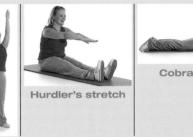

Hurdler's stretch

Cobra stretch

b: kick pump

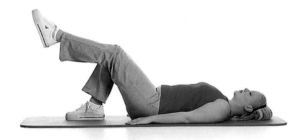

1 Now lie on your back with your arms resting at your sides. Bend your knees, and place your feet flat on your mat. Lift your left foot a few inches off the mat.

2 Exhale as you extend your left leg, stopping before you've locked your knee. Inhale, lower to the starting position, and repeat the move for 30 to 60 seconds. Now repeat with your right leg.

today's journal

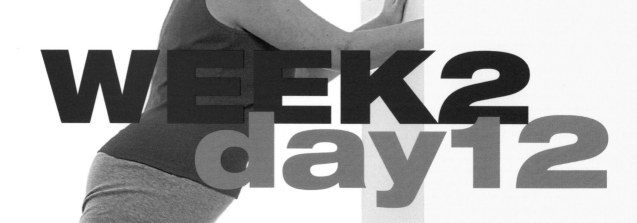

WEEK2
day12

> "*Never be afraid to ask a question, especially of yourself. Discovery is the mission of life.*"
>
> **Brian Kates**

the people solution

One of my favorite movies is the Academy Award–winning *Forrest Gump*. It's about a man who leads an extraordinary life even though he is handicapped. Forrest is able to make all his dreams come true because of how his mother taught him to see the world.

control the focus

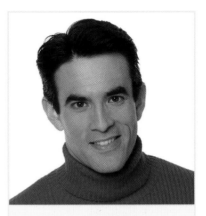

Forrest's mother explained things in a way that made Forrest ask what I call Result-Driven Questions (RDQs). Instead of asking himself, "Why am I disabled?" he asked questions such as, "Why did God make me so special?"

By asking Result-Driven Questions, you will not be able to focus on things that make you depressed or unmotivated. You have no option but to see things in a way that empower you. If you ask yourself and your inner team negatively driven questions such as, "Why is it so difficult for me to lose weight?" or "Why can't I lose weight?" or "What's my problem?" your answers will reveal all the reasons why you can't lose the weight. Using RDQs will give you the power to direct what you see and hear.

> "You need to read and think about the RDQs each and every day."

result-driven questions

Use these RDQs with yourself and your inner team every time you communicate. Photocopy this page and place it at your desk, or phone, or on your refrigerator so you see the questions often.

1. What joy will I feel when I attain my ultimate body?
2. How incredible will my life become when I am lighter?
3. What extraordinary things will people say to me when I am lighter?
4. How will I see my body shrink with the healthful choices I make?
5. What can I do today so that my weight-loss plans run smoothly?
6. How can I continue to create a weight-loss support network?

cruise moves
calves and butt

8-MINUTE LOG				
exercise	set 1	set 2	set 3	set 4
a				
b				

a: standing calf pump

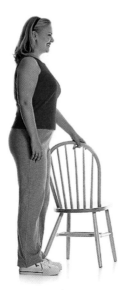

1 Stand next to a wall or sturdy chair with your feet directly under your hips and your arms resting at your sides. Check your posture.

2 Place one hand on the wall or chair for balance. Exhale as you rise onto the balls of your feet, bringing your heels off the floor. Inhale as you lower your heels back to the floor. Repeat for 60 seconds.

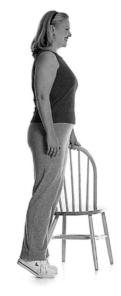

the cruise down plate: on-the-go meals

Many of my clients ask me what I think about meal replacement shakes and bars. I think they are excellent resources to use when you are extremely busy. According to the American Dietetic Association, meal replacement drinks and bars meet the demands of today's lifestyles for quick and easy dining and help you avoid high-fat, high-calorie choices from fast food chains. Of course, a regular Cruise Down Plate meal is always the best option, but sometimes it comes down to getting something fast (and healthy) or nothing at all. Make sure your drink or bar contains 300 to 400 calories. For more information on meal replacements, visit jorgecruise.com/onthegomeals.

exercise sequence

warm up

Jog or march in place.

cruise moves

Do one 60-second repetition of Cruise Move (a), then immediately

do one 60-second repetition of Cruise Move (b). Repeat this cycle 4 times, and you will be done in 8 minutes.

cool down

After your Cruise Moves, do these stretches (see page 107).

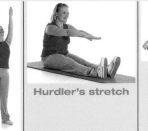

Sky-reaching pose

Hurdler's stretch

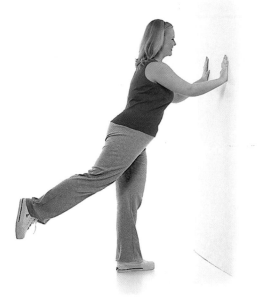

Cobra stretch

b: glute hold

Stand between 2 and 2½ feet in front of a wall. Place your palms against the wall with your elbows slightly bent. Lean into your palms for support. Then exhale and raise your right leg behind you as high as you can comfortably. Breathe normally as you hold for 30 to 60 seconds. Lower and repeat with your left leg.

today's journal

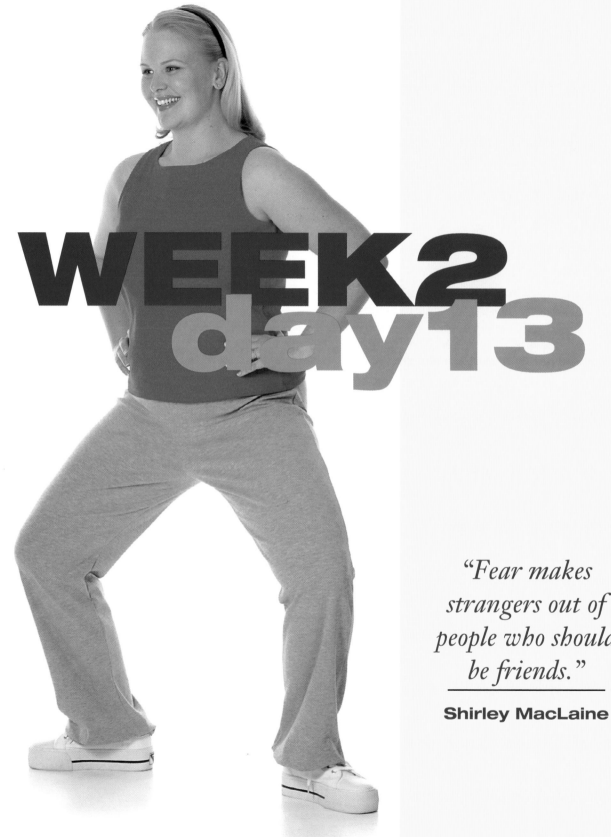

WEEK2
day13

"*Fear makes strangers out of people who should be friends.*"

Shirley MacLaine

the people solution

To avoid misunderstandings, sadness, and drama with your inner team, never make assumptions. I learned this when I read a book called the *The Four Agreements* by Don Miguel Ruiz. It's a lesson that has changed my life.

don't make assumptions

Simply put, you must always find the courage to ask questions and express what you really want. Don't assume that someone on your inner team understands that "it is important they call you back today" or "it is important that they e-mail you back today." If you need their support *today*, then find the courage to ask for what you need. Don't assume your team members know that you need them urgently. They cannot read your mind.

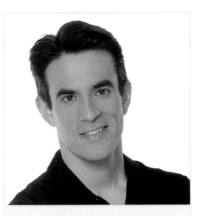

"Never make assumptions, and your communication with your inner team will be smooth."

cruise moves
inner and outer thighs

8-MINUTE LOG				
exercise	set 1	set 2	set 3	set 4
a				
b				

a: plié pump

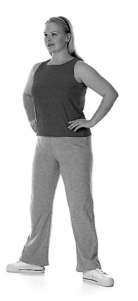

1 Stand with your feet as wide apart as you can comfortably place them. Point your feet like a duck. Place your hands on your hips, and check your posture.

2 Inhale as you bend your knees out to the sides and squat down as far as you comfortably can. Make sure your knees don't go out past your ankles. Exhale as you rise to the starting position. Repeat for 60 seconds.

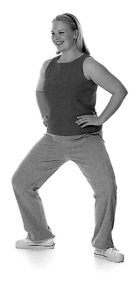

the cruise down plate: secrets for eating out

Don't let dining at a restaurant get in the way of your Cruise Down Plate eating system. Most restaurants serve huge portions of entrees and side dishes, and you don't want those extra calories lurking on your plate.

When you place your order, ask for a take-home container to be brought with your meal. When your dish comes, visualize your Cruise Down Plate and portion off the food on your plate accordingly. Anything that doesn't fit on

your plate in the allotted sections (unless they're veggies) goes into your take-home container. Without those extra morsels of temptation lurking about your plate, you'll be free to enjoy your meal without guilt!

exercise sequence

warm up

Jog or march in place.

cruise moves

Do one 60-second repetition of Cruise Move (a), then immediately

do one 60-second repetition of Cruise Move (b). Repeat this cycle 4 times, and you will be done in 8 minutes.

cool down

After your Cruise Moves, do these stretches (see page 107).

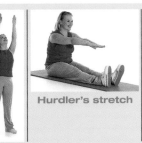

Sky-reaching pose

Hurdler's stretch

Cobra stretch

b: outer hold

Stand next to a wall or sturdy chair with your feet directly under your hips. Place your left hand against the wall or chair for balance, and place your right hand on your right hip. Exhale as you lift your extended right leg out to the side as high as you comfortably can. Hold for 30 to 60 seconds, breathing normally. Now repeat with the other leg.

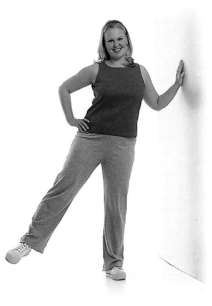

today's journal

WEEK 2
day 14

"No citizen has a right to be an amateur in the matter of physical training. . . . What a disgrace it is for a man to grow old without ever seeing the beauty and strength of which his body is capable."

Socrates

the people solution

It's time to record your second week's progress. This exercise will help to keep you focused and motivated. If you'd like to share your progress with me, send an e-mail with your answers to secondweek@jorgecruise.com.

capture your progress

Grab a pen and answer the following questions. Then share the answers with your accountability buddy. If you need more space, turn the page and continue writing in Today's Journal.

1. What is your current weight?

_____

2. What was your original weight?

_____

3. What have you done well this week? What makes you proud of you?

_____
_____
_____
_____
_____
_____

4. What could you improve next week?

_____
_____
_____
_____
_____
_____
_____

5. What is your game plan for week 3?

_____
_____
_____
_____
_____
_____
_____
_____

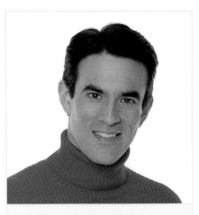

"I will e-mail you tips on how to make week 3 even more fun and effective."

cruise moves
your day off

Before I started Jorge's plan, I had stopped playing with my kids at the playground because my body couldn't take it. I had a hard time getting things done around the house because I was too tired.

> *"Now I can play with my kids, get everything done around the house, and teach my kids a healthy way to eat."*

I can tire my kids out, instead of getting tired out. After playing with my kids, I have enough energy to spend quality time with my wife, get my chores done, and still have time to relax!

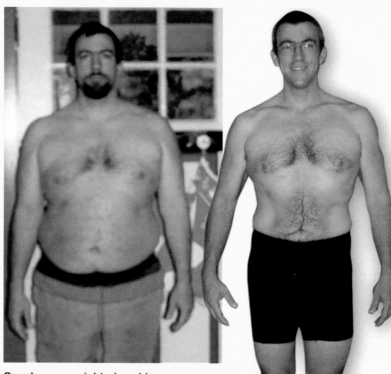

Sean's new weight gives him more energy.

the cruise down plate

When eating out, order extra vegetables with your meal. This will help to prevent you from filling up—and out— on higher calorie foods such as mashed potatoes and steak. But remember, while most vegetables are naturally low in calories, restaurants may add certain ingredients to them that suddenly turn them into high-calorie fare.

steamed veggies

To add flavor to vegetables, many restaurants sauté or fry them in heavy oils, cover them in rich sauces, or drench them in butter, all of which add lots of unwanted, artery-clogging saturated fat that can easily put you over your fat allowance for that meal.

To avoid this problem, order your vegetables steamed! You're not making an unreasonable request. Restaurants often specially prepare vegetables and other dishes without butter and sauce for people who have allergies or who are lactose intolerant (unable to tolerate dairy products). As a result, most restaurants will oblige your request, and you will be served piping hot, crisp, and ultra-nutritious and delicious veggies.

If you'd like to add your own bit of flavoring to punch up the taste, ask for a squeeze of lemon or lime juice, some chopped garlic, or a little balsamic vinegar, none of which will add calories to your meal. If you *want* to use your fat allotment on your veggies, then drizzle them with olive or flaxseed oil.

today's journal

WEEK3
day15

"*People are capable, at any time in their lives, of doing what they dream of.*"

Beth Bingham

the people solution

This week we will focus on People Solution secrets that will help you to further expand your buddy team. Adding a few more key people to your team will give you more flexibility and support.

talk 101

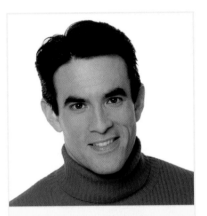

My clients often ask me how they can become better talkers, particularly when meeting new people. For example, they might see someone and want to ask, "You look so full of energy. What is your secret?" They want to be able to approach people and ask them about little things that will help to keep them motivated.

Here's the secret to successful talking: confidence. With confidence, you have a feeling of certainty that attracts others to you. What is the quickest way to feel more confidence? Good posture. When you stand tall, with your head up and shoulders back, you activate your diaphragm, changing your breathing. You inhale more oxygen, energizing your body. You feel more alive.

"This little secret will give you a major advantage when meeting and talking to people."

cruise moves
chest and back

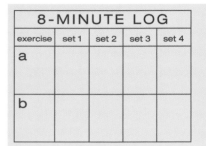

8-MINUTE LOG				
exercise	set 1	set 2	set 3	set 4
a				
b				

a: wall pump

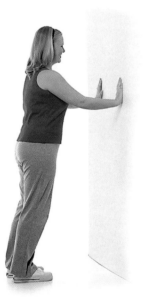

1 Stand at arms' length away from a wall with your feet directly under your hips. Lean forward and place your palms against the wall. Your elbows should be slightly bent.

2 Inhale as you slowly bend your elbows, bringing your chest and torso closer to the wall. Exhale as you slowly press yourself back to the starting position, straightening your arms as you go. Slowly repeat for 60 seconds.

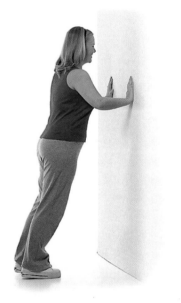

the cruise down plate: cook when you're not hungry

Cooking or baking for others can seem like a daunting task when you're following a weight-loss program, but you don't have to give in to the temptation that comes with it. If you need to bake cookies for a meeting, a cake for a birthday party, or dishes ahead of time for a dinner party, plan to do so during a time of the day when you're the least hungry. For many people, the morning is the time when their defenses are the strongest. You can also cook right after you've just had your largest meal of the day.

exercise sequence

warm up

Jog or march in place.

cruise moves

Do one 60-second repetition of Cruise Move (a), then immediately

do one 60-second repetition of Cruise Move (b). Repeat this cycle 4 times, and you will be done in 8 minutes.

cool down

After your Cruise Moves, do these stretches (see page 107).

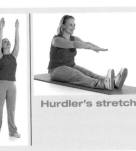

Sky-reaching pose

Hurdler's stretch

Cobra stretch

b: posture pump

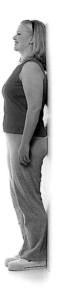

1 Stand with your heels, buttocks, and head against a wall or sturdy, closed door. Rest your arms comfortably at your sides.

2 Exhale as you pull your back and shoulders toward the wall, trying to flatten your entire upper back, from your ribs to your shoulders, against the wall. Try to get your lower back as close to the wall as you can. Relax and repeat for 60 seconds.

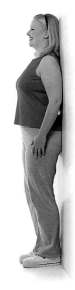

today's journal

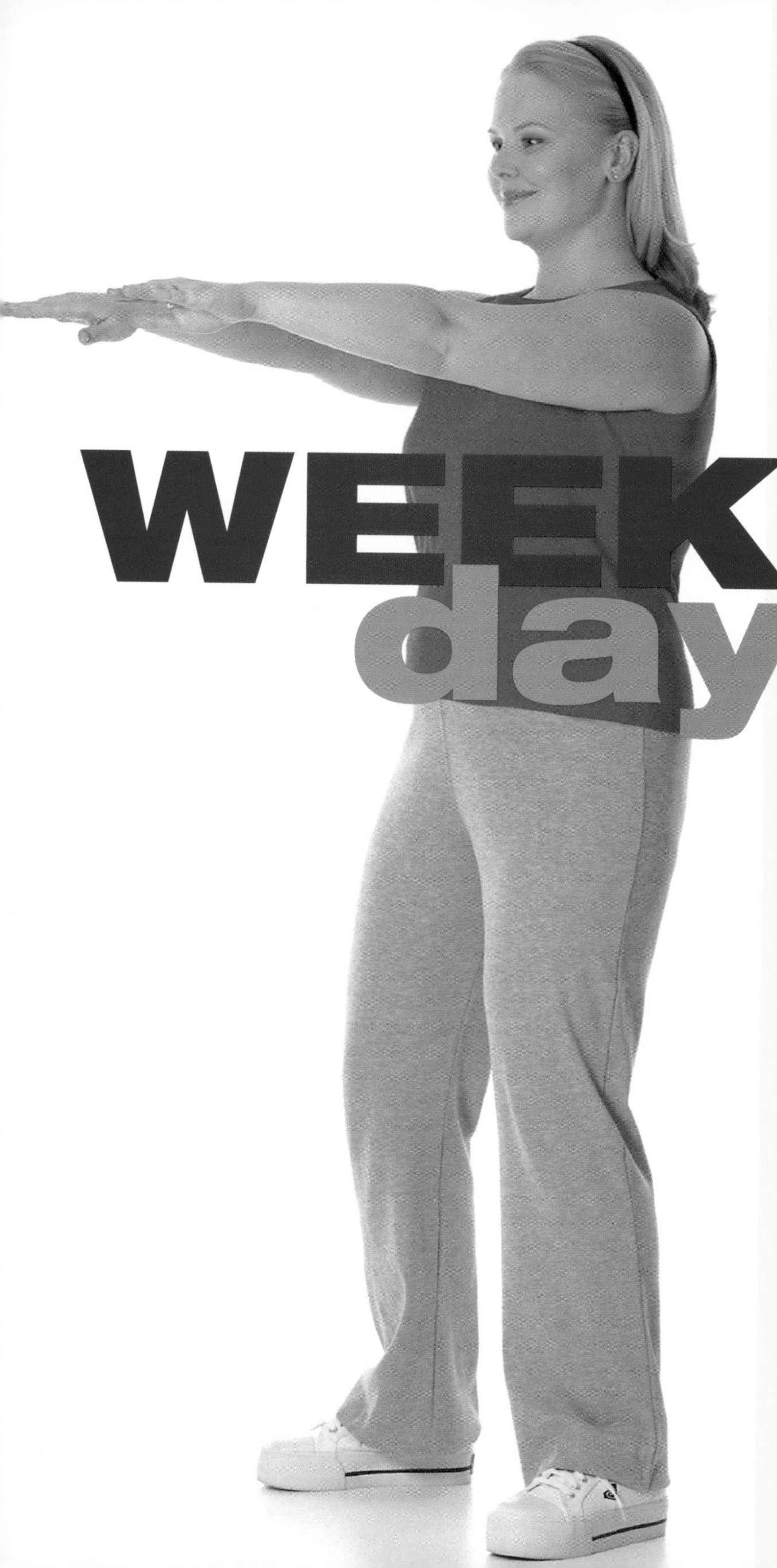

WEEK3
day16

"They can
because they
think they can."

Virgil

the people solution

Yesterday we talked about the power of confidence. So now that you have the confidence to help you meet new people, let's move on to what to say when you meet them. How do you break the ice?

ice breakers

Knowing how to start up a new conversation is critical. According to the best book ever written on this subject, *How to Win Friends and Influence People* by Dale Carnegie, the secret lies in genuine interest.

If you are going to approach a new person, you must have a genuine reason. Did you see this person ordering something delicious and you want to try the same dish? Does this person look as if he or she has so much energy, energy that you want to have? Those are genuine reasons. If you are speaking from your heart and genuinely want to talk to this person, you will always say the right thing.

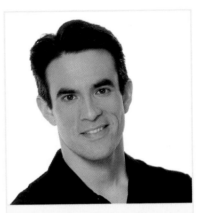

"Just be genuine, and almost anything you say to break the ice will be perfect."

cruise moves
shoulders and abdominals

8-MINUTE LOG				
exercise	set 1	set 2	set 3	set 4
a				
b				

a: sleepwalker hold

Stand with your feet directly under your hips, your abs firm, and your back long and straight. Exhale as you raise your arms in front of your torso to shoulder level. Hold for up to 60 seconds as you breathe normally. Make sure to keep your shoulders relaxed away from your ears.

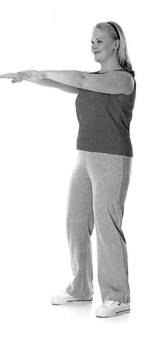

the cruise down plate: olive oil

Olive oil is composed of omega-9 fats, one of the good fats. As you can see from the super-market shelf, there are many olive oils from which to choose.

From regular to virgin to extra-virgin, here's what it all "oils" down to. Extra-virgin is the highest quality and hence, most expensive, olive oil on the market. To qualify as extra-virgin, the olives must have been picked at their optimum ripeness, giving the oil the richest flavor, and also the highest price tag. When a bottle is labeled just "olive oil," it contains some imperfections and lacks some of the rich flavor of the extra-virgin varieties. Obviously this olive oil is usually the least expensive on the shelf. Virgin olive oil falls somewhere in between extra-virgin and plain when it comes to taste, quality, and price. "Light" olive oil does not mean lighter in calories, but lighter in taste and appearance. If you don't like the strong taste of olive oil, go for the light variety.

exercise sequence

warm up

Jog or march in place.

cruise moves

Do one 60-second repetition of Cruise Move (a), then immediately

do one 60-second repetition of Cruise Move (b). Repeat this cycle 4 times, and you will be done in 8 minutes.

cool down

After your Cruise Moves, do these stretches (see page 107).

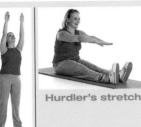

Sky-reaching pose

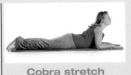

Hurdler's stretch

Cobra stretch

b: belly breath pump

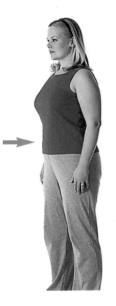

1 Stand with your feet directly under your hips. As you exhale, contract and press your tummy muscles in-ward as you slowly squeeze all the breath out of your lungs.

2 Reverse the motion by relaxing your tummy outward to slowly pull air into your lungs. Repeat for 60 seconds, breathing slowly, fully emptying and filling your lungs with the effort of your abdominals.

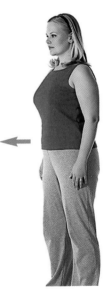

today's journal

WEEK3
day17

"*Loneliness and the feeling of being unwanted is the most terrible poverty.*"

Mother Teresa

the people solution

Yesterday I shared with you the power of genuine interest to break the ice during any conversation. Now you're ready for your final step in maximizing your ability to connect with strangers. Think of it as the cherry on top of the (low-calorie) ice-cream sundae.

the power of a smile

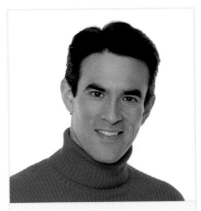

The cherry on top of your sundae is a smile. A smile says to people, "You make me happy. I like you." Your smile is a messenger that represents the good inside of you. It will dramatically improve your relationships with your buddies and yourself.

But your smile must come from deep inside. To make sure you show off a genuine smile, list 10 things that make you sincerely smile—things that you love and that bring true joy to you, such as a heartwarming memory, a funny joke, a baby's first step, and sunshine on your face. (If you need more space, turn the page and continue writing in Today's Journal.)

"Read your list whenever you need a prompt for your smile."

10 things that make me smile

1. _____
2. _____
3. _____
4. _____
5. _____
6. _____
7. _____
8. _____
9. _____
10. _____

cruise moves
triceps and biceps

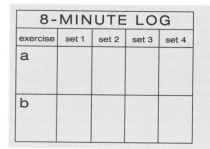
a: kickback can pump

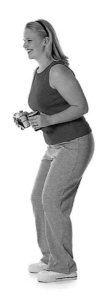

1 Stand with your feet directly under your hips. Bend forward from your hips about 45 degrees. Grasp a soup can in each hand. Bend your arms 90 degrees, keeping your upper arms pressed against your torso.

2 Exhale as you press your hands up past your torso, keeping your upper arms against your sides. Stop once you've extended your arms. Inhale as you lower. Repeat for 60 seconds.

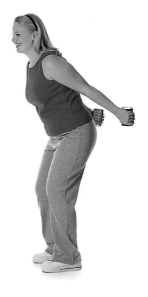

the cruise down plate: a ziploc baggie

Buying your food in bulk will save you a bunch of cash. But be careful not to lose your portion control amidst the jumbo bulk bags and boxes. Here's one tip: Never eat straight from the food container. Don't bring the huge bag of nuts or giant box of crackers to the couch to munch from while you're watching TV. Instead, measure out your portion in the kitchen and put it in a bowl. Then put the food away—and keep it there. That way you won't unconsciously eat more than you had planned.

You can also measure out several portions and seal each one individually in small Ziploc bags. When you need to grab a snack in a hurry, you won't have to spend the time measuring. You can just grab a baggie and hit the road. Remember, there are no bad food choices, just bad portion sizes.

exercise sequence

warm up

Jog or march in place.

cruise moves

Do one 60-second repetition of Cruise Move (a), then immediately

do one 60-second repetition of Cruise Move (b). Repeat this cycle 4 times, and you will be done in 8 minutes.

cool down

After your Cruise Moves, do these stretches (see page 107).

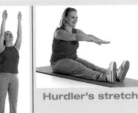

Sky-reaching pose

Hurdler's stretch

Cobra stretch

b: curl can pump

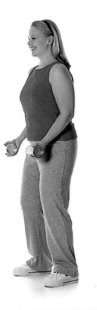

1 Stand with your feet directly under your hips. Grasp a soup can in each hand. Rest your arms at your sides, palms and soup cans facing forward, with a slight bend in your elbows.

2 Exhale as you raise the soup cans toward your upper arms. Stop about 45 degrees before the cans reach your upper arms. Inhale as you return to the starting position. Repeat for 60 seconds.

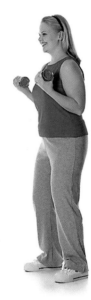

today's journal

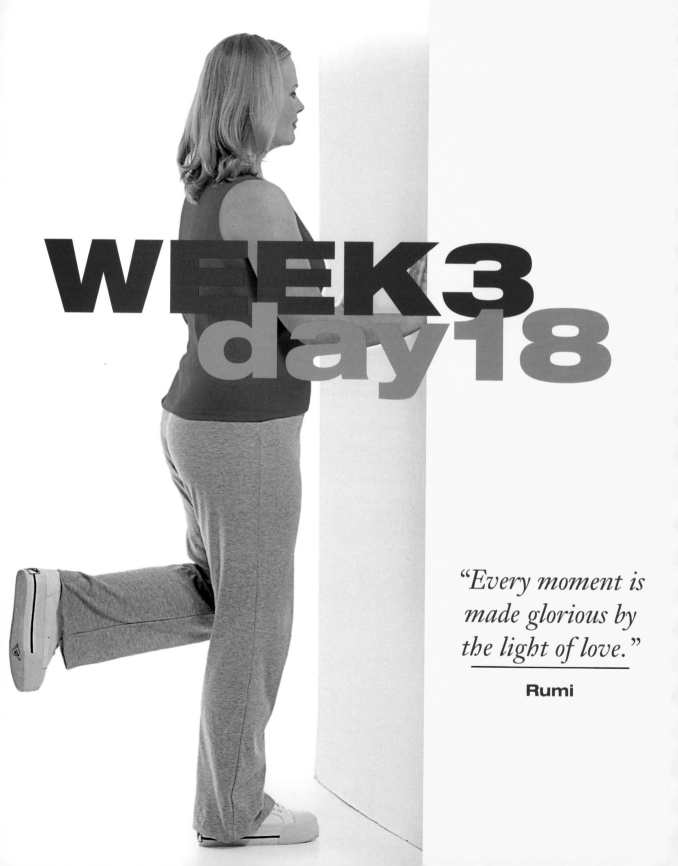

WEEK3
day18

> *"Every moment is made glorious by the light of love."*
>
> **Rumi**

the people solution

You have already read countless stories shared by my clients. In chapter 3, you read some of the painful and distressing stories that led many of them to overeat.

share your story

My clients first told me many of these stories online on the message boards at JorgeCruise.com. Doing so helped remove an emotional weight from their shoulders. They received countless messages of support and friendship from people on the site. They heard from strangers saying that they had been through the same thing and that they understood what they had gone through. Before long, their online relationships developed into friendships, and their buddy teams expanded.

The more people you have to listen to you and nurture you, the easier your weight loss will become. Visit www.jorgecruise.com and share your story on our message boards. You will meet some wonderful new people who really care.

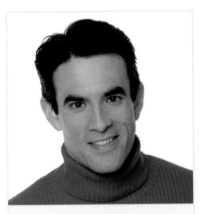

"Sharing your story will transform your life."

cruise moves
hamstrings and quadriceps

a: lift pump

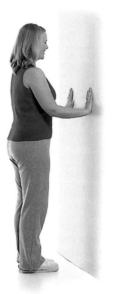

1 Stand about 1 foot in front of a wall with your feet directly under your hips. Rest your hands against the wall for balance. Check your posture.

2 Exhale as you lift your left foot toward your left buttock. Stop once you achieve a 90-degree angle. Inhale, lower, and repeat this move for 30 to 60 seconds. Then repeat with your right leg.

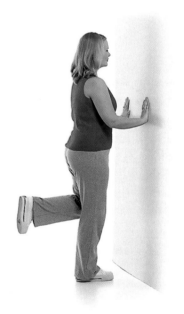

the cruise down plate: nibbles count

Many people tell me that they hardly eat anything at all but still can't manage to lose weight. I ask them if they ever nibble on samples of food at the grocery store or dip into the candy dish at work. Those little calories that most people like to think of as "freebies" can actually be the culprit of some serious weight gain. Without knowing it, your spoonfuls of soup to taste, nibbles of bread, samples of ice-cream flavors, and handfuls of jelly beans can add up to 100 extra calories a day. That could amount to an extra 10 pounds per year! So if you take a nibble here and there, don't forget that it's a part of your daily food allowance. There are no such things as food freebies!

exercise sequence

warm up

Jog or march in place.

cruise moves

Do one 60-second repetition of Cruise Move (a), then immediately

do one 60-second repetition of Cruise Move (b). Repeat this cycle 4 times, and you will be done in 8 minutes.

cool down

After your Cruise Moves, do these stretches (see page 107).

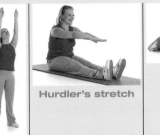

Sky-reaching pose

Hurdler's stretch

Cobra stretch

b: squat pump

1 Stand with your feet directly under your hips. Place your hands on your hips. Check your posture.

2 As if you were sitting into an imaginary chair, inhale as you bend your knees and squat so that your knees are bent no more than 90 degrees. (Only squat as deeply as you feel comfortable.) Make sure your knees remain over your ankles (not out past your toes). Keep your abdominals firm and back straight as you squat. Exhale as you press up to the starting position. Repeat for 60 seconds.

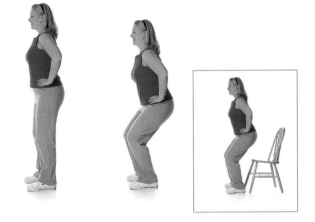

If you worry about falling back, place a chair behind you and literally squat until your butt touches the chair.

today's journal _____

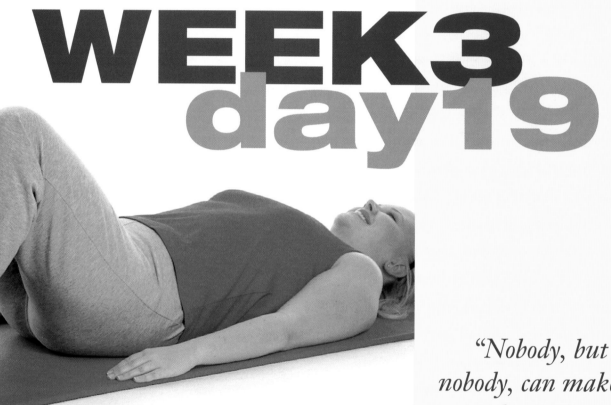

WEEK3
day19

> *"Nobody, but nobody, can make it out here alone."*

Maya Angelou

the people solution

I learned from my good friend and mentor, Anthony Robbins, that change is automatic. It's an inevitable part of life. It's a given that our physical bodies will change as we age, that our financial status will change, that our relationships with others will change, and that our jobs will change. But progress only comes from conscious thought, decisions, and actions. Change is automatic, but progress is not.

weekly online meetings

That is why I invite you to attend weekly online meetings with a weight-loss mentor at JorgeCruise.com. My mentors will help you to uncover ideas that can save you months of time, energy, or frustration. The mentors are friends, motivational speakers, and weight-loss coaches—all in one. They are very special people that not only have worked with me personally but also have walked the talk. They have successfully lost weight the Jorge Cruise way. They know what you're going through because they've been there.

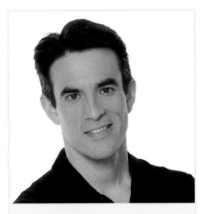

"Change is automatic, but progress is not."

cruise moves
calves and butt

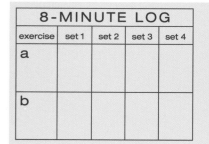

8-MINUTE LOG				
exercise	set 1	set 2	set 3	set 4
a				
b				

a: tippy toe pump

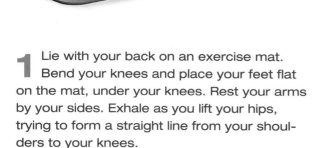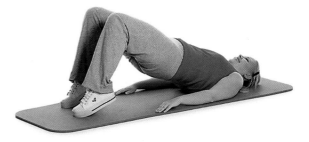

1 Lie with your back on an exercise mat. Bend your knees and place your feet flat on the mat, under your knees. Rest your arms by your sides. Exhale as you lift your hips, trying to form a straight line from your shoulders to your knees.

2 Inhale, then exhale again as you raise your heels off the mat as high as you can. With your hips still raised, inhale as you lower your heels, then exhale and lift, repeating the sequence for 60 seconds.

the cruise down plate: avoid the bad fat trap

Remember that all fats are not created equal, and saturated and trans fats are the worst for you. Saturated fats and trans fat (hydrogenated fats) make the body produce more cholesterol, which may raise blood cholesterol levels and increase your risk of heart disease. So it is very important to lower your intake of these unhealthy fats. One way to do this is to switch from red meat such as beef to white meat such as turkey or chicken. White meat contains 33 to 80 percent less fat than red meat.

exercise sequence

warm up

Jog or march in place.

cruise moves

Do one 60-second repetition of Cruise Move (a), then immediately

do one 60-second repetition of Cruise Move (b). Repeat this cycle 4 times, and you will be done in 8 minutes.

cool down

After your Cruise Moves, do these stretches (see page 107).

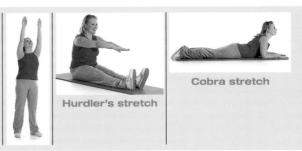

Sky-reaching pose

Hurdler's stretch

Cobra stretch

b: lift-up hold

While still lying on the floor, bend your knees and place your feet flat on the floor. Exhale as you lift your hips as high as you can, trying to form a straight line from your shoulders to your knees. Hold for up to 60 seconds as you breathe normally.

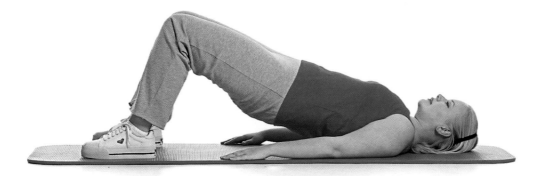

today's journal

WEEK3
day20

"The first step
towards getting
somewhere is to
decide that you are
not going to stay
where you are."

J. P. Morgan

the people solution

Remember the story I shared with you about Sharon, Edna, and Cheryl in chapter 3? They were part of a San Diego "Jorge Cruise" book club. The club started with 25 regular attendees and grew and grew.

create your own book club

Look in your local Yellow Pages and find the top three bookstores. Then call the stores and ask for the name of the person who arranges book clubs. E-mail, call, or visit that person and hatch your idea to start a club. As I said in chapter 3, the store manager will most likely help you to promote the club. You can't go wrong.

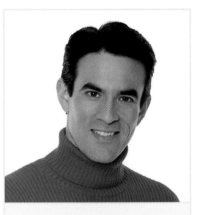

"A book club can help reinforce your growing network of buddies."

cruise moves
inner and outer thighs

8-MINUTE LOG				
exercise	set 1	set 2	set 3	set 4
a				
b				

a: plié hold

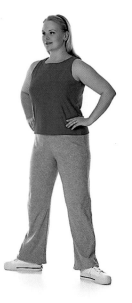

1 Stand with your feet as wide apart as you can comfortably place them. Point your feet like a duck. Place your hands on your hips, and check your posture.

2 Inhale as you bend your knees out to the sides and squat as far as you comfortably can. Make sure your knees don't go out past your ankles. Hold for 60 seconds.

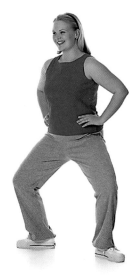

the cruise down plate: sugarless gum

If you're a person who loves to chew gum while you drive or suck on hard candy while you work, you still can! Just make sure that you do so with sugarless varieties of gum and hard candy. A sweet tooth doesn't mean that your weight-loss program is doomed. Just be conscious of what type of sweets you choose. A stick of regular gum can add 10 extra calories and candy as much as 20 calories apiece. This might not sound like a big indulgence, but if you chew on five sticks of gum a day and suck on five hard candies, you could be taking in 150 useless calories! So be sure to stick with sugarless versions of these types of sweets, and you'll keep your weight loss on target.

exercise sequence

warm up

Jog or march in place.

cruise moves

Do one 60-second repetition of Cruise Move (a), then immediately

do one 60-second repetition of Cruise Move (b). Repeat this cycle 4 times, and you will be done in 8 minutes.

cool down

After your Cruise Moves, do these stretches (see page 107).

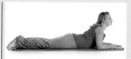

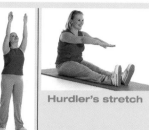

Sky-reaching pose

Hurdler's stretch

Cobra stretch

b: outer pump

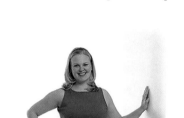

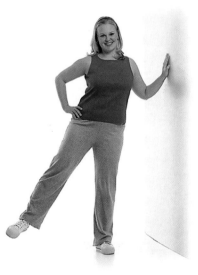

1 Stand next to a wall or sturdy chair with your feet directly under your hips. Place your left hand against the wall for balance, and place your right hand on your hip. Shift your weight over your left foot as you raise your right foot slightly off the floor.

2 Exhale as you lift your right leg out to the side as high as you comfortably can. Inhale as you lower. Repeat for 30 to 60 seconds. Then switch sides.

today's journal

WEEK 3
day 21

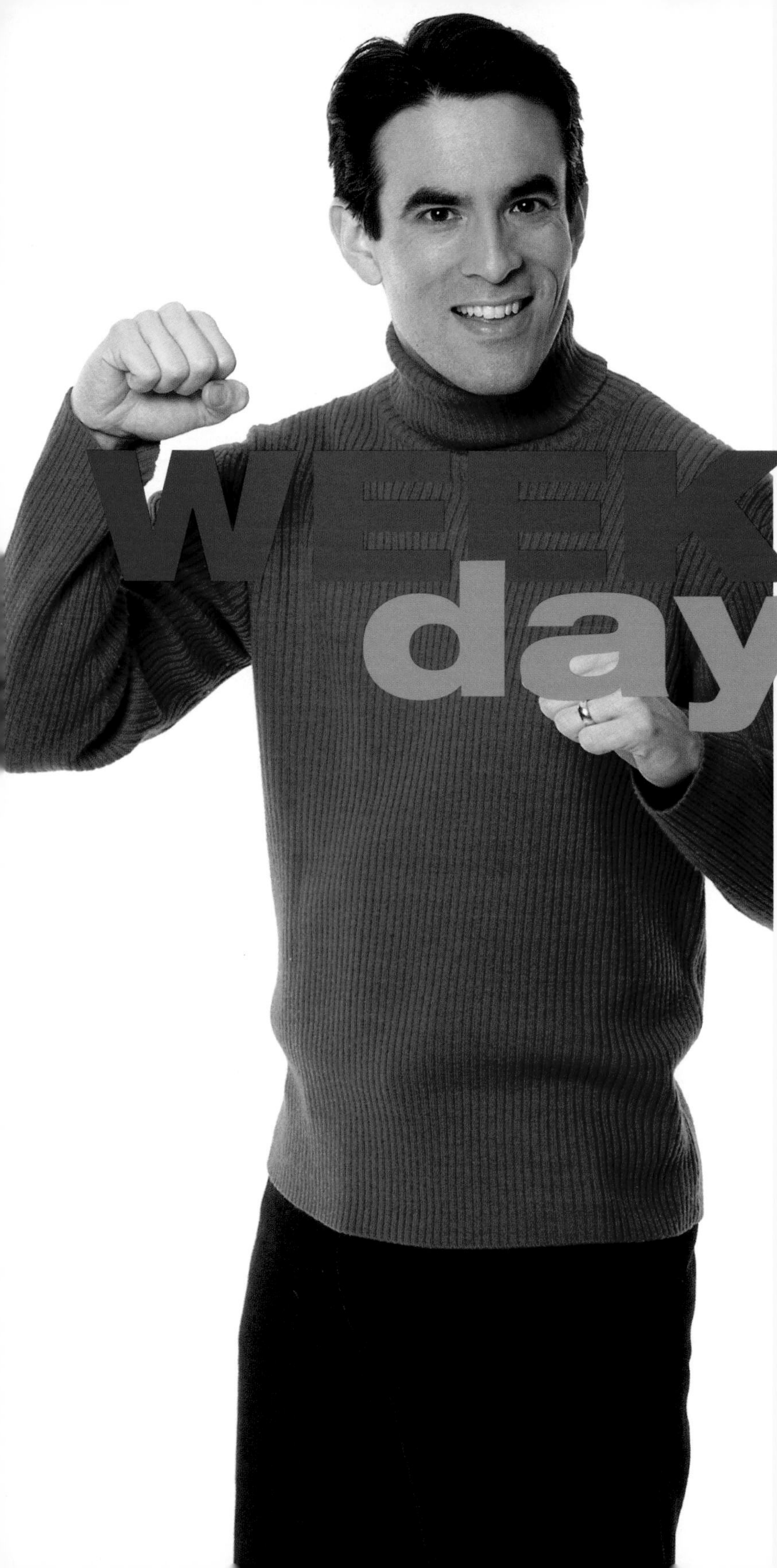

"If you put everything off until you're sure of it, you'll get nothing done."

Norman Vincent Peale

the people solution

It's time to record your third week's progress. This will help to keep you focused and motivated. If you'd like to share your progress with me, send an e-mail with your answers to thirdweek@jorgecruise.com.

capture your progress

Grab a pen and answer the following questions. Then share this with your accountability buddy. If you need more space, turn the page and continue writing in Today's Journal.

1. What is your current weight?

_____

2. What was your original weight?

_____

3. What have you done well this week? What makes you proud of you?

_____
_____
_____
_____
_____
_____
_____

4. What could you improve next week?

_____
_____
_____
_____
_____
_____
_____

5. What is your game plan for week 4?

_____
_____
_____
_____
_____
_____
_____

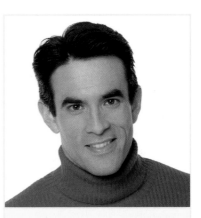

"I will e-mail you bonus tips on how to make week 4 even more fun and effective."

cruise moves
your day off

Before Jorge's plan, I was always out of breath. I mean always, even while tying my shoes, doing housework, walking. I hated going anywhere that required me to wear nice clothes.

"Even though some still consider me to be overweight, I feel so good about myself now."

I know I have a much better chance of being here when my son finishes school, gets married, and has children of his own. With this program, I have proved to myself that I can be healthy and live a very fulfilling life.

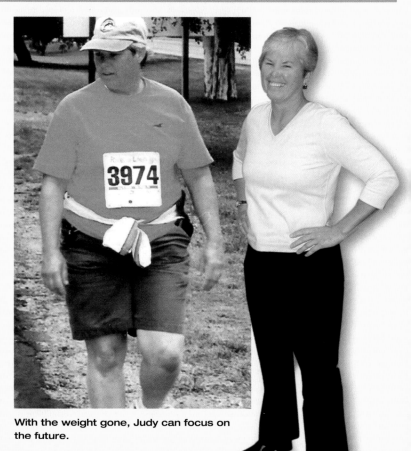

With the weight gone, Judy can focus on the future.

the cruise down plate

Bread doesn't have to be a guilty pleasure, as long as you eat the right type of bread. Whole-grain bread is packed with fiber and slow-release carbohydrates, which will keep your insulin levels stable. When you're shopping for whole-grain bread, don't be fooled by misleading packaging. Just because the bread looks dark in color does not mean it is whole grain. Make sure you read the label and see that it says, "100% whole grain" or "100% whole wheat." Breads that are only labeled as "wheat" might be refined, which is not what you want.

the best bread

A close second to 100 percent whole-grain bread is sourdough. Though it does not come packed with the same amount of fiber, sourdough is slightly acidic, causing your digestive tract to slowly break it down and release it into your bloodstream.

If you're making bread at home, consider adding ground flax seeds to your favorite recipe. The seeds will add fiber, health-promoting lignans, and healthful fats to your bread. They'll also help slow down digestion and suppress your appetite for the rest of the day.

today's journal _____

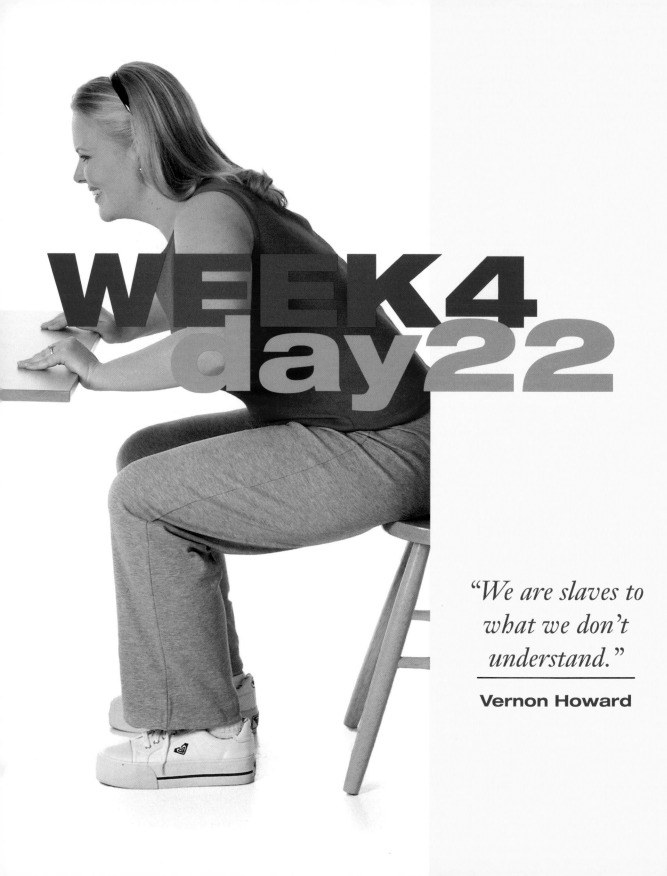

WEEK4
day22

> "*We are slaves to what we don't understand.*"
>
> **Vernon Howard**

the people solution

This week I will share with you resources that will maintain your ongoing success. The resources include everything from books, magazines, and Web sites to music and even electronic gadgets.

empowering books

Today I will share some of my favorite books. Books can provide wonderful information, inspiration, and guidance. They have the power to change your life, as they are often the product of many years of study and experience from experts passionate about their topics.

In my office I keep a quote from Erasmus, one of the greatest scholars of all time, who lived during the Renaissance: "When I get a little money, I buy books; and if any is left, I buy food and clothes." My favorite books include:

• *If Life Is a Game, These Are the Rules* by Chérie Carter-Scott, Ph.D.

• *How to Win Friends and Influence People* by Dale Carnegie

• *The Seat of the Soul* by Gary Zukav

• *Think and Grow Rich* by Napoleon Hill

• *The Four Agreements* by Don Miguel Ruiz

• *Awaken the Giant Within* by Anthony Robbins

• *How to Talk to Anyone, Anytime, Anywhere* by Larry King

• *Life's Little Emergencies* by Emme

• *Sexy at Any Size* by Katie Arons

• *Fast Food Nation* by Eric Schlosser

• *Flax for Life!* by Jade Beutler

• *Understanding Fats and Oils* by Michael T. Murray, N.D., and Jade Beutler

• *Brilliant Food Tips and Cooking Tricks* by David Joachim

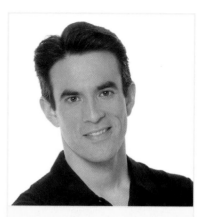

"Add as many books to your weight-loss library as possible."

• *Eating Well for Optimum Health* by Andrew Weil, M.D.

• *Eat Up, Slim Down* by Jane Kirby

• *The Human Body Explained* by Philip Whitfield

• *Sleep Disorders* by Herbert Ross, D.C.

cruise moves
chest and back

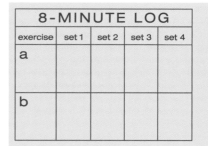

8-MINUTE LOG				
exercise	set 1	set 2	set 3	set 4
a				
b				

a: table pump

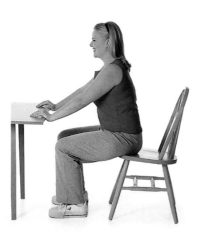

1 Sit on the edge of a sturdy chair 2 to 3 feet in front of a table. Place your palms on the tabletop with your arms extended.

2 Inhale as you bend your elbows and lean forward from your hips, bringing your chest toward the table. Once you can no longer bend forward, exhale as you press back to the starting position. Repeat for 60 seconds.

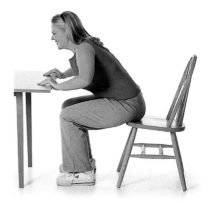

the cruise down plate: fast food restaurant secrets

Just because your busy schedule forces you to eat fast food some of the time, your diet doesn't have to suffer. Remember, no foods are off-limits. It's portion control that matters. But fast food restaurants these days are not in the business to help you lose weight; they're in the business to give you a bigger portion than the next chain for less money. Stay away from all "supersize" deals. In many cases, your best bet might be the child-sized portion, which is actually quite a normal-sized meal. Also, be sure to order a diet soda or ice water so you're not adding an additional 200 calories just from your beverage.

exercise sequence

warm up

Jog or march in place.

cruise moves

Do one 60-second repetition of Cruise Move (a), then immediately

do one 60-second repetition of Cruise Move (b). Repeat this cycle 4 times, and you will be done in 8 minutes.

cool down

After your Cruise Moves, do these stretches (see page 107).

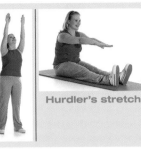

Sky-reaching pose

Hurdler's stretch

Cobra stretch

b: pull-down hold

Sit 2 to 3 feet in front of a table in a sturdy chair with your feet flat on the floor. Bend forward and extend your arms, placing your palms against the tabletop. Exhale as you press down onto the table. Hold firmly for 60 seconds as you breathe normally.

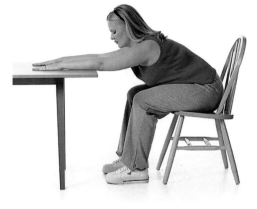

today's journal

WEEK4
day23

"*The body is a marvelous machine . . . a chemical laboratory, a power-house. Every movement, voluntary or involuntary, full of secrets and marvels!*"

Theodore Herzl

the people solution

A magazine subscription is one of the best gifts you can give yourself and others. Each magazine offers great ideas and inspirational photos. They can be a wonderful source of encouragement and information. Each magazine sets you up to win!

motivational magazines

Today, check out some of the best health and lifestyle magazines at the newsstand or in a bookstore. Eventually, I want you to subscribe to one or two of these magazines for monthly inspiration. If you have a favorite magazine that is not on my list below, e-mail your suggestion to magazines@jorgecruise.com. My favorite magazines include:

- *Cooking Light*
- *Dr. Weil's Self-Healing Newsletter*
- *First for Women*
- *Fitness*
- *Men's Health*
- *Organic Style*
- *O, The Oprah Magazine*
- *Prevention*
- *Psychology Today*
- *Quick Cooking*
- *Self*
- *Shape*

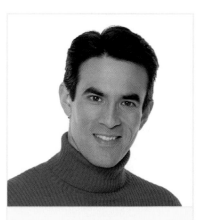

"Each magazine sets you up to win!"

cruise moves
shoulders and abdominals

8-MINUTE LOG				
exercise	set 1	set 2	set 3	set 4
a				
b				

a: roller coaster pump

1 Stand with your feet directly under your hips, your abs firm, and your back long and straight. Exhale as you raise your arms in front of your torso to shoulder level.

2 Lower your arms to the starting position as you inhale.

3 Exhale as you raise your arms out to your sides. Stop once they reach shoulder height, then inhale and lower them to the starting position. Repeat the entire sequence for 60 seconds.

the cruise down plate: the best vitamin supplement

Because your Cruise Moves cause a small breakdown in your muscle fibers, you may need a vitamin C supplement to help your lean muscle tissue recover more quickly. My favorite brand is Emergen-C. Emergen-C is a little packet of powder that you pour into a glass of water. Just stir it up and you will have a fizzy, delicious beverage that is packed with 1,000 milligrams of vitamin C, 28 different minerals, and various B vitamins. It's caffeine-free, but all those vitamins will make you feel ready to charge.

exercise sequence

warm up

Jog or march in place.

cruise moves

Do one 60-second repetition of Cruise Move (a), then immediately

do one 60-second repetition of Cruise Move (b). Repeat this cycle 4 times, and you will be done in 8 minutes.

cool down

After your Cruise Moves, do these stretches (see page 107).

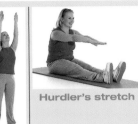

Sky-reaching pose

Hurdler's stretch

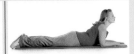

Cobra stretch

b: belt hold

Stand with your feet slightly wider than hip-width. Lengthen your spine and relax your shoulders. Then exhale as you pretend someone is tightening a belt or corset around your waist and midsection. Pull in and tighten your abdominals. Hold them in this position as you breathe normally for up to 60 seconds.

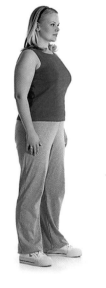

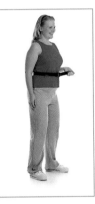

today's journal

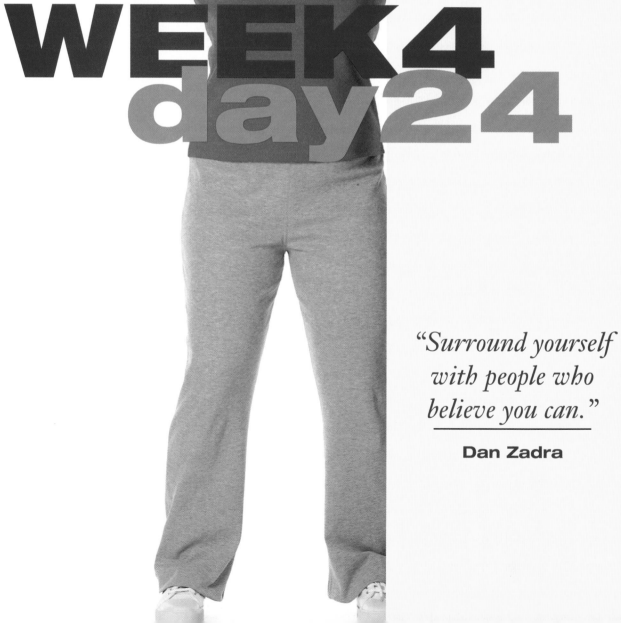

WEEK4
day24

"*Surround yourself with people who believe you can.*"

Dan Zadra

the people solution

As you know, I have built my whole weight-loss career around the Internet, and I truly believe the Internet is one of the most powerful tools in today's world. Web sites allow us instant access to other people for support, the latest news on health and weight-loss trends, easy shopping, and great healthy cooking recipes.

wonderful web sites

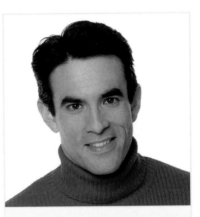

"I truly believe the Internet is one of the most powerful tools in today's world."

Try to visit at least three weight-loss Web sites today. If you find a great site that I've missed, e-mail it to websites@jorgecruise.com. Check out this list of my favorites:

- www.anthonyrobbins.com
- www.webmd.com
- www.ivillage.com
- www.miguelruiz.com
- www.oprah.com
- www.oxygen.com
- www.zukav.com
- www.diabetes.org
- www.drweil.com
- www.eatright.org
- www.prevention.com
- www.betternutrition.com
- www.acefitness.org
- www.acsm.org
- www.ideafit.com
- www.kathysmith.com
- www.jacklalanne.com
- www.pureenergies.com
- www.vectrafitness.com
- www.powerblock.com
- www.clubone.com
- www.crunch.com
- www.brevail.com
- www.jorgecruise.com

cruise moves
triceps and biceps

8-MINUTE LOG				
exercise	set 1	set 2	set 3	set 4
a				
b				

a: kickback hold

Stand with your feet directly under your hips. Bend forward from your hips about 45 degrees with your arms extended behind you, toward the floor. Exhale as you lift your extended arms behind your torso. Stop once you've extended your arms, but before you've locked your elbows. Hold for 60 seconds.

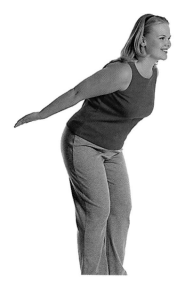

the cruise down plate:
salad toppings and dressings

You probably know that you must avoid many salad toppings in order to lose weight. But did you know that some toppings are low-calorie and tasty? Avoid deli meat cubes, which can add up to 100 calories and 6 grams of fat for just 8 to 10 little pieces. In-stead, reach for the beans, like kidney or garbanzo. These beans are virtually fat-free, loaded with good-for-you vitamins such as folate, and very tasty. Instead of the bacon bits, add sunflower seeds, a great source of magne-sium. Use crumbled flavored rice cakes instead of oily croutons. As for dressings, stay away from the creamy varieties such as ranch and thousand island, and instead add a tablespoon of an oil-based vinaigrette. Or try my favorite—drizzle a tablespoon of flaxseed oil over your salad.

exercise sequence

warm up

Jog or march in place.

cruise moves

Do one 60-second repetition of Cruise Move (a), then immediately

do one 60-second repetition of Cruise Move (b). Repeat this cycle 4 times, and you will be done in 8 minutes.

cool down

After your Cruise Moves, do these stretches (see page 107).

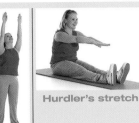

Sky-reaching pose

Hurdler's stretch

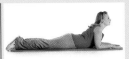

Cobra stretch

b: "show off my muscle" hold

Stand with your feet slightly wider than your hips. Firm your abdominals, lengthen and straighten your back, and relax your shoulders. Raise your arms out to the sides, with your palms facing up. Curl your hands in loose fists toward your shoulders. Once in position, show off that muscle! Firm and flex your biceps and hold for 60 seconds.

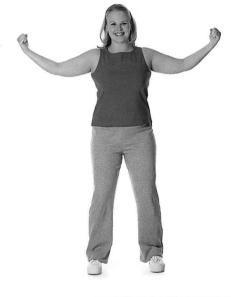

today's journal

WEEK4
day25

> "Death is not the greatest loss in life. The greatest loss is what dies inside us while we live."
>
> **Norman Cousins**

the people solution

To become your own greatest friend, you must know how to motivate and inspire yourself to move forward and succeed. Today I am going to share with you my secret weapon to making your morning Cruise Moves routine even more fun. It centers on the power of music.

the magic of music

Music improves your Cruise Moves simply because it adds energy and emotion. And with more energy and emotion, you can do anything! Get out your CD player and start listening to music that makes you feel great. Listen to your inspirational tunes in the morning when you do your Cruise Moves. You can even go to www.jorgecruise.com/music to hear selections from my personal picks of the most inspiring and moving music.

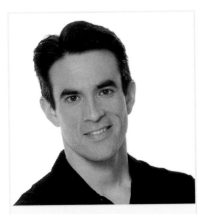

"Music improves your Cruise Moves simply because it adds energy and emotion."

cruise moves
hamstrings and quadriceps

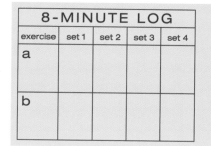

8-MINUTE LOG				
exercise	set 1	set 2	set 3	set 4
a				
b				

a: ham lift hold

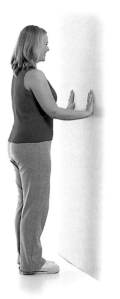

1 Stand about 1 foot in front of a wall with your feet directly under your hips. Rest your hands against the wall for balance. Check your posture.

2 Exhale as you lift your left foot toward your left buttock. Stop once you achieve a 90-degree angle. Hold for 30 to 60 seconds as you breathe normally, then switch legs.

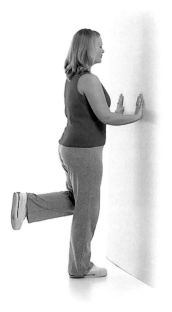

the cruise down plate: avocado power

Avocados have gotten an unfair bad rap due to their high-fat content. For starters, avocados contain beta-sitosterol, which helps inhibit cholesterol absorption from the intestines, re-

sulting in lower blood cholesterol levels. They also contain glutathione, an antioxidant that research has linked to the prevention of heart disease and various types of cancers, in-

cluding cancer of the mouth and pharynx. So go ahead and dip into the guacamole. Count it as your fat serving for that meal.

exercise sequence

warm up

Jog or march in place.

cruise moves

Do one 60-second repetition of Cruise Move (a), then immediately

do one 60-second repetition of Cruise Move (b). Repeat this cycle 4 times, and you will be done in 8 minutes.

cool down

After your Cruise Moves, do these stretches (see page 107).

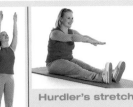

Sky-reaching pose

Hurdler's stretch

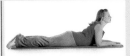

Cobra stretch

b: wall hold

Stand with your feet directly under your hips and your head, shoulders, and back against a wall. Slowly walk your feet forward as you bend your knees, sliding downward along the wall as far as you can without bringing your knees past your ankles or your buttocks below your knees. Hold for 60 seconds as you breathe normally.

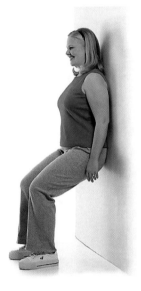

today's journal

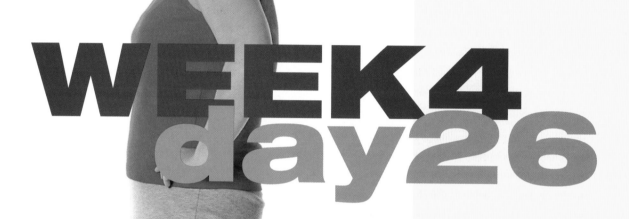

WEEK4
day26

> *"Life shrinks or expands in proportion to one's courage."*
>
> **Anaïs Nin**

the people solution

Today I want to share with you five of my favorite tools that I personally use to make weight loss fun.

cool hi-tech gadgets

My favorite gadgets include:

Freestyle's The Buzz watch. You can set the watch alarm to vibrate every 3 hours to help you to remember to eat. Find out more at www.freestyleusa.com.

Apple's iPod. I use this to listen to my music anywhere I go. What is an iPod? It's an MP3 player that holds 1,000 songs and can go with you wherever you go. Plus it works with both PCs and Macs. Check it out at www.apple.com.

Nike's PSA Play 128 Max. If you want a smaller, lighter MP3 player, my next favorite is Nike's PSA Play 128 Max. It holds fewer songs than the iPod, but it's lighter and designed for movement. Find out more at www.nike.com.

BodyGem. By simply breathing into this little hand-held device for a few minutes you can know precisely how many calories your body burns in a day. It is a great way to compare your "before" metabolism with your "after" metabolism. It's available for sale to qualified wellness advisors only, but many local gyms will have one that you can use. To find out more or to find a facility near you, visit www.healthetech.com.

Tanita Body Fat Monitor/ Scale. This is the scale I use at home (on Sundays). I recommend it to all my clients. It can store your weight each week and compare it for you, plus it can also tell you your percentage of body fat. Bottom line: It is a great way to see more of your success and will keep motivated. Find out more at www.tanita.com.

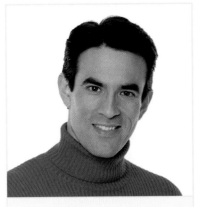

"These gadgets can help make weight loss fun!"

cruise moves
calves and butt

8-MINUTE LOG				
exercise	set 1	set 2	set 3	set 4
a				
b				

a: high-heel hold

Stand with your feet directly under your hips.
Exhale as you lift your heels, rising onto the
balls of your feet. Pretend you are wearing
very high heels. (Place one hand on a sturdy
chair or wall for balance.) Hold for 60 seconds.

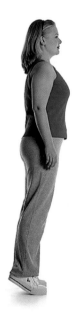

the cruise down plate: dairy

The protein in dairy products, called casein, is an allergen that can cause asthma and sinus problems. I can vouch for that; as soon as I cut most of the dairy out of my diet, my headaches and asthma symptoms went away. Some people's digestive tracks can't process the sugar, or lactose, in dairy products. If you love to pour milk on your cereal and eat sandwiches with cheese, try switching to soy products. For every dairy product you can think of, there is a soy substitute. There are soy versions of milk, cheese, sour cream, butter, yogurt, and even ice cream. They don't taste exactly like the real thing, but sometimes, they taste even better.

exercise sequence

warm up

Jog or march in place.

cruise moves

Do one 60-second repetition of Cruise Move (a), then immediately

do one 60-second repetition of Cruise Move (b). Repeat this cycle 4 times, and you will be done in 8 minutes.

cool down

After your Cruise Moves, do these stretches (see page 107).

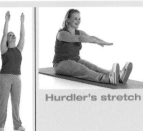

Sky-reaching pose

Hurdler's stretch

Cobra stretch

b: pelvic tilt pump

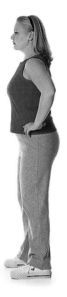

1 Stand with your feet directly under your hips and your hands on your hips. Check your posture.

2 Exhale as you curl your tailbone forward and down, your pubic bone up, and your belly button in, tilting the top of your pelvis back and the bottom of your pelvis forward. Inhale as you relax. Repeat for 60 seconds.

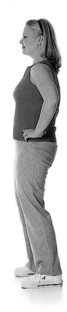

today's journal

WEEK4
day27

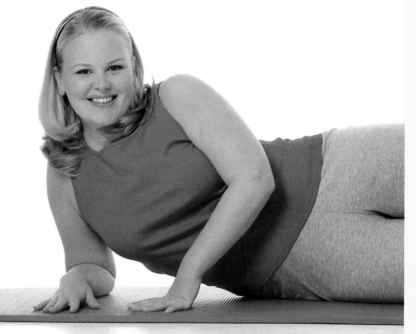

*"The greatest waste
in the world is
the difference
between what we
are and what
we could become."*

Ben Herbster

the people solution

When you look through your old photo albums, do you feel the emotions captured in the photos? Imagine a special birthday, wedding, or graduation photo. Can you put yourself back at that moment and feel it again? Photographs can move us to feel a certain way almost instantly.

create some eye candy

Photos can also motivate you to do your Cruise Moves. Have you ever seen someone in great shape and thought, "I want to look like that," then found yourself doing your next set of moves with more excitement and motivation?

Start creating an Eye Candy Collage. Here's how it works: Flip through three or four magazines and cut out five or more photos of people who are healthy and fit. Or you might use photos of you when you were at a healthier weight. Cut them out and paste them onto a piece of poster board. Put your Eye Candy Collage in a place where you will see it throughout the day.

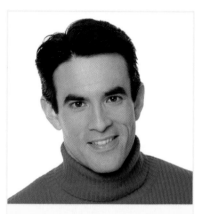

"Use your Eye Candy images to fuel your motivation to move."

cruise moves
inner and outer thighs

a: inner circles pump

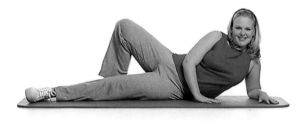 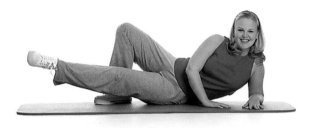

1 Lie on an exercise mat on your left side with your legs extended. Support your body weight on your left forearm. Rest your right hand on the mat in front of your tummy for support.

2 Bend your right knee and place your right foot on the mat behind your left leg. Lift your extended left leg about 1 foot off the mat. Then hold the lift and draw clockwise circles with your left foot for 30 to 60 seconds. Relax and repeat with your right leg.

the cruise down plate: juice caution

Fruit juice is loaded with vitamins and antioxidants that can improve your health. But most types are also loaded with calories. If you love juice and want its nutritional goodness but don't want the calories, dilute it. Fill your glass halfway with sparkling water and the rest of the way with your favorite juice. You can add sparkling water to everything you drink, from wine to tomato juice and even soda.

exercise sequence

warm up

Jog or march in place.

cruise moves

Do one 60-second repetition of Cruise Move (a), then immediately

do one 60-second repetition of Cruise Move (b). Repeat this cycle 4 times, and you will be done in 8 minutes.

cool down

After your Cruise Moves, do these stretches (see page 107).

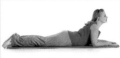

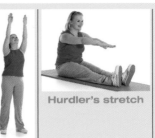

Sky-reaching pose

Hurdler's stretch

Cobra stretch

b: outer circles pump

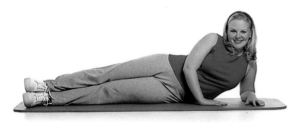 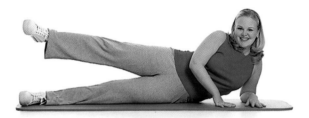

1 While still lying on the mat on your left side with your legs extended, support your body weight on your left forearm. Rest your right hand on the mat in front of your tummy for support.

2 Lift your extended right leg about 1 foot off the mat, above your left leg. Draw clockwise circles with your right foot as you hold the lift for 30 to 60 seconds. Lower and repeat with your left leg.

today's journal

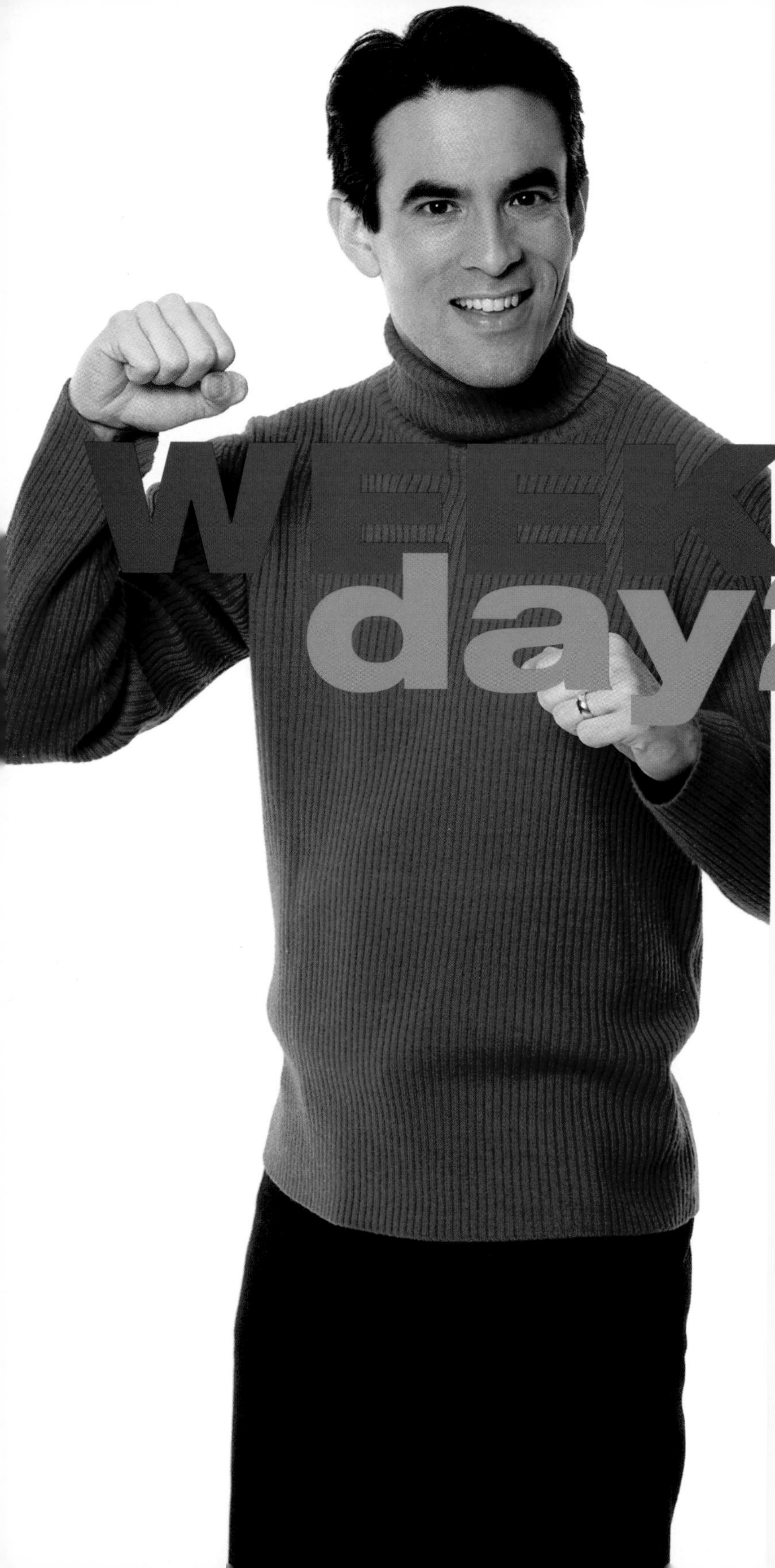

WEEK 4
day 28

"I've failed over
and over and over
again in my life.
And that is why
I succeed."

Michael Jordan

the people solution

It's time to record your fourth week's progress. This will help to keep you focused and motivated.

capture your progress

Grab a pen and answer the following questions. Then share this with your accountability buddy. If you need more space, turn the page and continue writing in Today's Journal.

1. What is your current weight?

_____

2. What was your original weight?

_____

3. What have you done well this week? What makes you proud of you?

_____
_____
_____
_____
_____
_____

4. What could you improve next week?

_____
_____
_____
_____
_____
_____
_____

5. What is your game plan for next week?

_____
_____
_____
_____
_____
_____
_____
_____

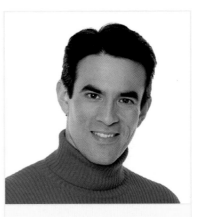

"Share your progress with me by e-mailing your answers to fourthweek@ jorgecruise.com."

cruise moves
your day off

Before Jorge's plan, I felt frustrated with my unhealthy eating habits and lack of a regular exercise routine. My common sense told me "good food in moderation, lots of water and exercise" were the three keys to healthy, permanent weight loss, but with two young boys to care for, it was always a battle to get to the gym on a consistent basis. Since discovering Jorge Cruise's program, I literally roll out of bed and, in my pajamas, do my moves before my day has even begun!

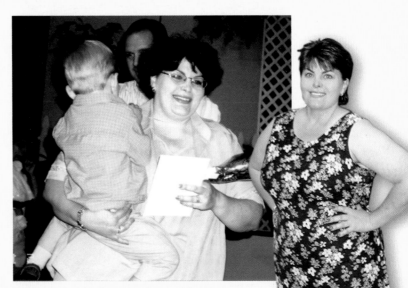

Robin moves in the morning and feels great all day.

"By exercising first thing in the morning, I make better food choices throughout the day and drink more water."

I no longer go to bed each night feeling like a failure, but instead I feel excited for a new day. Talk about starting off each day with a positive step. This program is my answer for life!

the cruise down plate

If you're like many of my clients, you love butter. Most people don't want to give it up. The good news is that there is room for all foods on the Cruise Down Plate, including butter. I want you, however, to try a simple switch for a few days.

a word about butter

Fill a small plastic container with olive oil and place it in your refrigerator. The oil will solidify, taking on the consistency of butter. Just spread ½ tablespoon of this on your toast instead of butter. It will taste different at first, but after a few days, your taste buds will grow used to it.

You can also use olive oil as a "dip." Just drizzle a bit into a shallow dish. Then dip small pieces of bread into the oil. Use extra-virgin oil for more flavor. To increase the taste of your oil "dip," add freshly chopped garlic or dried spices such as salt, pepper, or oregano. Or, consider trying a preflavored oil, such as garlic-flavored olive oil.

Of course, as I said, there is room for all foods on the Cruise Down Plate. When you want to use butter, go right ahead. Just make sure to stick to your fat allowance.

today's journal _____

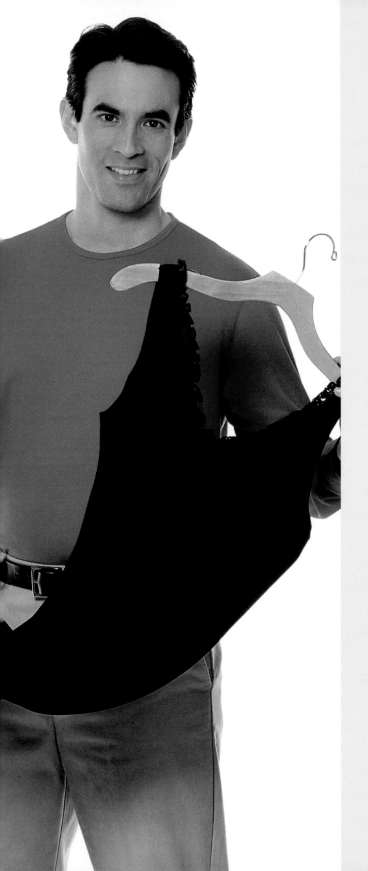

8
Your New Life

How to Maintain Your Success or Lose Even More Weight

beyond the first 28 days

You have just completed your first 28 days on the *8 Minutes in the Morning for Real Shapes, Real Sizes* weight-loss plan. Great job and congratulations on your success so far!

stay successful

In my introductory letter, I told you that you would get hooked on this way of living. You've invested your energy and effort in making better choices that have helped you lose weight. You made choices that will keep you feeling and looking great forever. Keep up the great work!

This chapter is all about keeping you successful. In the following pages, you'll learn how to lose more weight (if that's your goal) and how to keep the weight off. I've left no questions unanswered. When you're done reading, you will know exactly what to do to keep losing more. And just as important, once you lose the 30 or more pounds, you will find out how to keep it off for life!

how to lose more

During your first 28 days on my *8 Minutes in the Morning for Real*

Shapes, Real Sizes plan, you should have lost about 8 to 10 pounds. To lose a total of 30 pounds, you must follow the program for two additional 28-day cycles. If you have more than 30 pounds to lose, then you will keep following the same 28-day cycle until you reach the weight-loss target date you wrote on page 45 in chapter 3. It's that simple.

Each day you will continue to do The People Solution activities. Repetition is the mother of all skills. Each time you do The People Solution activities, you will become better at them. It's like listening to a new song. The more you hear it, the better you remember the words. Eventually you can hear it in your head without actually listening to the music. It becomes yours. That's my goal in having you repeat The People Solution activities. Eventually, The People Solution will become so ingrained in your life that you no longer need a prompt to put it into action.

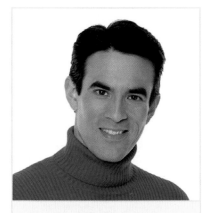

"Know that there will be some weeks that you might not drop as many as 2 pounds. That's okay."

In addition to The People Solution activities, each day you will continue to do your Cruise Moves. Your Cruise Moves provide the key to permanently boosting your metabolism by firming and strengthening your muscles.

And last but not least, after your 8 minutes each day, continue to use the Cruise Down Plate eating system. Reread my tips each day to fully ingrain them into your lifestyle.

It's that simple. I know you will do great!

what to do if you plateau

After the first 2 or 3 months on the program, some of you might hit a small plateau.

First, relax and stay positive. Know that there will be some weeks that you might not drop as many as 2 pounds. That's okay. Many of you might just lose 1 pound. That is still great progress, so don't beat yourself up.

During your first 4 weeks on the program, you probably lost 1 to 2 pounds a week like clockwork. After a few months, however, it's not uncommon for weight loss to move at a slightly slower pace. Every once in a while you might lose less than 2 pounds. And every once in a while you might lose no weight at all that week. That's okay. You've just hit a temporary plateau. Chances are that your body is still burning fat but your weight on the scale has remained

stagnant due to other factors, such as fluid bloating.

If you have stuck with every aspect of my plan, then you are doing your best. Be patient with your body and stay on course. Don't ever give up. Don't get distressed or discouraged.

You will break through your plateau if you stay focused on what you want. Remember that focus is power. Make sure that you are using your Cruise Down Plate and Cruise Weight-Loss Planner. Double-check that you are eating at the right times, and keep doing your Cruise Moves in the morning. And, of course, continue to eliminate emotional eating by using The People Solution.

Plateaus almost always result from feeling discouraged and then overeating to lift your spirits. So seek extra support and nurturing to break through your plateau. Reach out to your inner team. Go online to JorgeCruise.com and chat with others about the program. Enlist the support of a weight-loss mentor at an online weekly meeting.

Here's another tip for avoiding plateaus that I learned from one of my most successful clients, Tina Draney. When she hit her first plateau, she wrote a detailed essay titled "What the Extra-Fat Is Costing Me." She e-mailed me

a copy, and I was so inspired that I asked if I could share it with you. Tina replied, "Absolutely!" She told me, "Looking at what the extra fat cost me in so many areas of my life was a wake-up call. If I ever plateau, I read this essay to remind me what life was like back then."

You can read her essay on page 225. I recommend you write your own essay to read whenever you hit a plateau. It will help to keep you motivated.

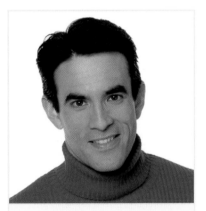

"I hope you will continue to think, move, and eat in this way for the rest of your life."

how to keep the weight off

Once you reach the target date you wrote on page 45, I truly hope that you will continue to follow the program. Why? This new lifestyle will have become such a part of your life that you won't want to quit. You will continue to think, move, and eat in this way for the rest of your life.

For example, my weight-loss mentors who run the various meetings at JorgeCruise.com are people who have successfully lost weight using all the principles in this book. They all continue to use the plan to maintain their success. They continue to think, move, and eat the Jorge Cruise way.

So go ahead and stick with the program long after you've reached your goal weight. I hope you'll continue to do your Cruise Moves each morning for the rest of your life!

But there are two caveats. Eventually, as your muscles get firmer and stronger, you may need a more challenging Cruise Moves routine. In that case, it may be time for you to graduate to the more advanced moves found in my first *8 Minutes in the Morning* book. You can find that book online and at all bookstores.

Second, if your weight drops *below* your ideal weight, then you must modify your Cruise Down Plate eating system. To do so, *double your snacks* each day. You can do this in a number of ways. For example, try one of the following methods:

• Instead of eating two snacks each day, have four.

• When it's time for a snack, double your snack serving size.

• Eat an additional snack along with lunch and dinner.

tina draney lost 32 pounds

It's a good thing I committed to Jorge's program, or I might officially be a hermit by now. Before I began the program, I spent more time hiding out in my house than getting out and enjoying life. I wore baggy shirts and sweatpants. I was just existing as an unhealthy and unsatisfied person.

> "Shopping for clothes used to be traumatic, but now it's fun."

Now that I've lost more than 30 pounds, I am amazed at that change in the shape of my body. I replaced my entire wardrobe. It's now full of color.

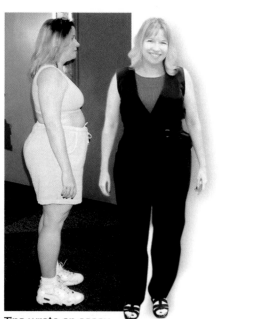

Tina wrote an essay to help maintain her success.

TINA'S PLATEAU-BUSTING WORDS OF WISDOM

One of my clients, Tina Draney, wrote an essay, excerpted here,
to read whenever she hit a plateau.

"When I look down at my chest, stomach, legs, I don't look so big. Then I see myself in a mirror. I find it hard to believe it is really me. Still, it doesn't seem to be bad enough for me to take massive action. *The extra fat costs me my reality.*

"I cringe whenever I'm asked to be in a picture. I hide behind others so my overweight body won't appear in the photo. *The extra fat costs me my self-respect.*

Since I've ballooned to my current size, I tend to hide myself from others. Most of the input I make to conversation is intellectual. I rarely add wit or playful conversation. I stay conservative and almost uptight because I don't want to draw attention to myself. *The extra fat costs me my personality and liveliness.*

I'm concerned about my health. My cholesterol is very high. I worry that my teeth might rot from my highly acidic, sugary diet. I don't like the appearance of my skin. My muscles are weak and I'm horribly flabby. *The extra fat costs me my health and appearance.*

I go through stages of binging. Usually it starts with a trigger—something at work or in my day that is unsettling. It's as if another person is inside begging me to stop eating, but usually she doesn't win the argument. Sometimes it seems as if I'm forcing myself to overeat to punish myself. *The extra fat costs me my self-control and a lot of money on food.*

I desire to be with a man who is fit, sexy, and athletic. I want him to be confident with a high level of self-esteem and high standards for himself. I know I can't attract this type of man when my body is in such bad shape and my self-esteem is so lacking. *The extra fat costs me the man of my dreams.*

I lack energy. Often I have stomachaches, headaches, heartburn, and a host of other uncomfortable sensations. I can sleep eight hours and still wake up tired. After a heavy meal in the evening, I'll wake up feeling hungover. *The extra fat costs me my energy and vitality.*"

WALK THIS WAY

Once you've reached your goal weight, consider adding power walking to your Cruise Moves. It will help to reduce stress and improve your overall health. I recommend you *always* do your Cruise Moves in the morning because they provide your most effective weight-loss solution, and fit in power walking when you have more time and when you want to strengthen your heart and melt away stress.

To get started, walk until you get out of breath or start to tire, then return home. Note how long your first walk took, and then build from there, increasing your time no more than 10 percent each week. For optimal heart protection, work up to 25 or 30 continuous minutes of walking.

Work on adding duration first. Then, once you can walk continuously for 25 to 30 minutes, begin to push the pace. You should never pant, however, and your legs should never hurt. If you feel either, you are walking too fast or too far for your fitness level. Back off a little and then slowly add distance or intensity. If you rate your effort on a scale of 1 to 10 (with 1 feeling easy and 10 feeling hard), it should fall somewhere between 6 and 8. That's your fat-burning zone. You'll feel better in that zone as well as reap the most benefits from your exercise.

tips from cruisers

To help you maintain your success, I asked my clients for their best tips in sticking to the program for life. This is what they told me.

• "Concentrate on how you feel, not the weight you lost or didn't lose. During my third month, there was a week where I didn't lose weight. I looked at the scale and felt my heart sink. Eventually, I began to see this miniplateau as a way to concentrate on other successes, such as my renewed energy, smaller clothing size, or being able to keep the weight off."
—Anne Armstrong

• "Every day, journal about anything that is on your mind. Write down your thoughts to remind yourself about what you are most grateful for."
—Erin McLeod

• "Don't leave the house without a snack. You might find yourself stuck somewhere and feel tempted to eat unhealthy foods."
—Ann Kirkendall

• "If you slip up, don't give yourself permission to keep doing it. Instead, stop, reevaluate your progress, forgive yourself, and start the program again."
—Bonnie Barrett

• "Don't eat until you've done your Cruise Moves. My motivation for getting my moves done in the morning is that I won't let myself eat anything until I've finished them."
—Lynnette Perkins

• "Always be prepared. Have veggies on hand so you can grab and munch on them whenever you are hungry."
—Melissa Winegar

• "Make a list of things to do instead of eating. That way, whenever an emotion triggers you to reach for food, you can consult your list and instead read, go for a walk, call a friend, take a bubble bath, and so on."
—Jeanna Erickson

Many of my clients also told me that they place their Power

Pledge Poster all over the house—particularly in the kitchen—to remind themselves of their goals and dreams. Others said that focusing on drinking plenty of water (one glass each hour), eating every 3 hours, and using flaxseed oil to curb their appetites were among the most important strategies for following the Cruise Down Plate and Cruise Moves for life.

I wholeheartedly thank you for allowing me to be your friend and weight-loss coach. I hope you will mail me your story and "before" and "after" photos so I can acknowledge you and possibly even feature you in my next book, on my TV appearances, or at JorgeCruise.com. You can find my office mailing address, phone numbers, and e-mail address at www.jorgecruise.com/contact.

I wish you all the best. I know you will do it. *Congratulations!*

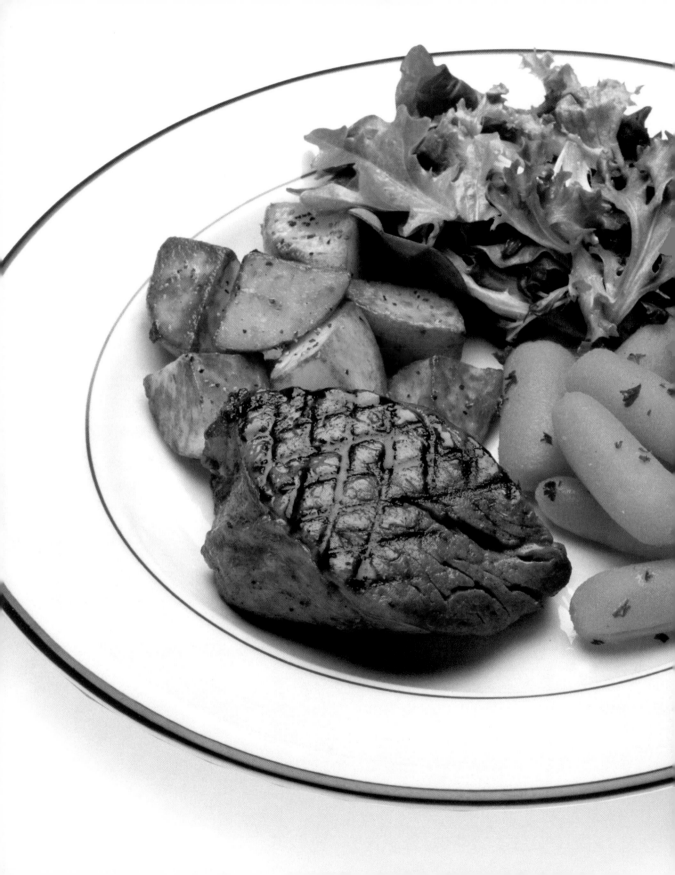

4

Beyond the 8 Minutes

9

The Easy Way to Use the Cruise Down Plate

a sample week of easy eating

If you're still not quite sure how to use the Cruise Down Plate, you'll find everything you need to know right here.

simple and delicious

For help on figuring out how to place foods on the plate in the correct portions, I've started you off with a sample week of Cruise Down Plate meals. Just follow the photos on pages 233–39 for 1 week, and you'll automatically get on track. Just remember: These are optional samples. To follow the Cruise Down Plate, you need only follow one simple rule: Fill half the plate with vegetables and the other half with equal portions of carbohydrate and protein foods, along with a tablespoon of fat. And if you are still hungry, have another plate of vegetables. It's that easy!

Use these photos and menus for ideas and inspiration. You may substitute any sample meal for another. For example, if you like a breakfast from day 2 and want to use it again on day 7, that's fine. And don't forget that you can spice up all of these meals with any seasoning or condiment from my "freebies" list on page 245. Enjoy, and eventually you'll be creating your own delicious Cruise Down Plates in the right portions for weight loss. For even more help on ensuring you fill your plate with the right portions, check out my food lists on pages 240–45.

critical secrets

Follow one simple rule for the Cruise Down Plate: Fill half your plate with vegetables, a quarter of your plate with carbohydrate foods, a quarter of your plate with protein foods, and use one tablespoon of fat.

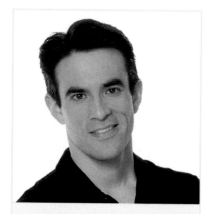

"If you are still hungry, have another plate of vegetables."

Day 1

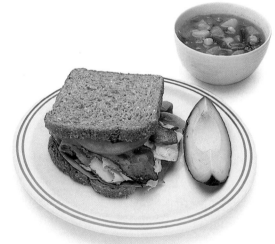

Breakfast 1 cup milk with ½ cup Uncle Sam Cereal; ½ grapefruit; 12 almonds

Snack 3 celery sticks filled with 1 teaspoon peanut butter each

Lunch Sandwich (2 reduced-calorie slices of bread, 2 ounces turkey, 1 slice lean bacon, lettuce, sliced tomatoes); ¼ avocado; 1 cup vegetable soup

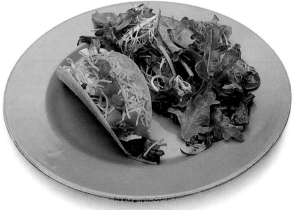

Snack 30 raisins

Dinner Taco (2 ounces lean ground beef, 6-inch corn tortilla, 1 ounce fat-free shredded cheese, shredded lettuce, diced tomatoes, salsa); mixed green salad with 1 tablespoon flaxseed oil

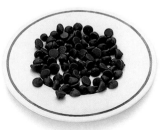

Treat ½ tablespoon chocolate chips

Day 2

Breakfast 6 scrambled egg whites; 1 small potato, cubed and sautéed in 1 tablespoon olive oil; 1 orange

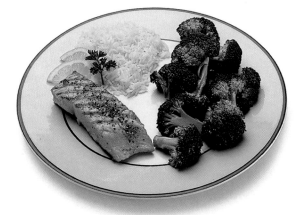

Snack 1 string cheese stick

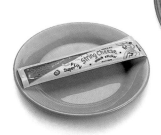

Lunch Taco salad (2 ounces ground turkey taco meat, 1 ounce fat-free shredded Cheddar cheese, 15 crumbled fat-free baked tortilla chips, 2 tablespoons oil-based salad dressing, shredded lettuce, diced tomato, onions, carrots)

Snack 1 cup air-popped popcorn sprinkled with Mrs. Dash seasoning

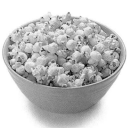

Dinner 3 ounces grilled salmon; ½ cup basmati rice; half-plate broccoli with 1 tablespoon flaxseed oil

Treat 1 Reese's Peanut Butter Cup

Day 3

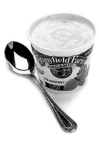

Breakfast 1 cup milk; ½ cup oatmeal; ¾ cup blueberries; 12 walnuts

Snack 8 ounces low-fat yogurt

Lunch Sandwich (3 ounces canned tuna mixed with 1 tablespoon reduced-calorie mayo and stuffed into half a 6-inch pita along with lettuce and tomatoes); 1 cup tomato soup

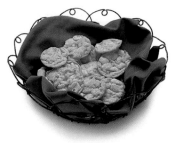

Snack 25 Soy Crisps

Dinner Chicken "sausage" pasta (2 ounces sliced chicken sausage, ½ cup whole wheat pasta, ½ cup marinara sauce); mixed green salad with 2 tablespoons oil-based salad dressing)

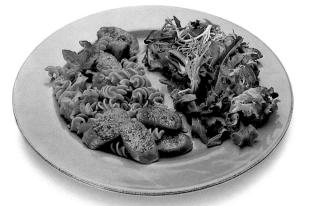

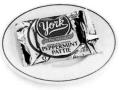

Treat York peppermint pattie

Day 4

Breakfast Veggie omelet (6 egg whites mixed with lots of veggies); ½ bagel with 2 tablespoons reduced-fat cream cheese; ⅓ cup juice-packed pineapple chunks

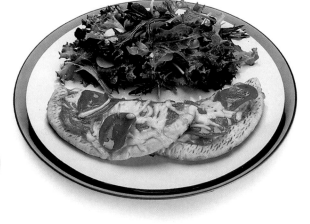

Snack 12 cashews

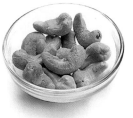

Lunch Pita pizza (1 ounce fat-free mozzarella, 2 ounces sliced turkey pepperoni, tomato sauce on 6-inch pita); mixed green salad with 1 tablespoon flaxseed oil and chopped fresh garlic

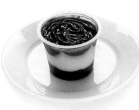

Snack Fat-free pudding cup

Dinner "Fried" chicken (3 ounces chicken rolled in bread crumbs and baked); ½ cup mashed potatoes with 1 tablespoon olive oil; steamed veggies

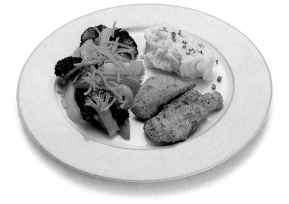

Treat 3 gingersnaps

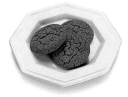

Day 5

Breakfast 3 slices lean bacon; 2 4-inch pancakes with 1 cup sliced strawberries, 1 tablespoon reduced-calorie butter, and 2 tablespoons sugar-free syrup

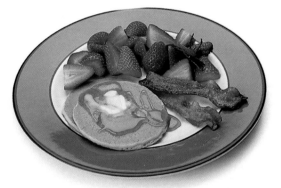

Snack Low-fat granola bar

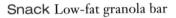

Lunch 1 sushi California roll (rice, crabmeat, cucumber, avocado, seaweed); 1 cup miso soup

Snack 1 piece peanut brittle

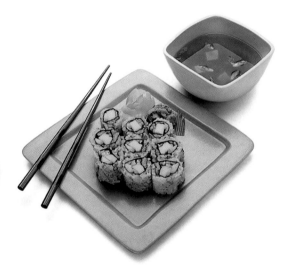

Dinner "Meat and potatoes" (3 ounces lean steak served with ½ cup roasted red potatoes); steamed carrots; mixed green salad with 1 tablespoon flaxseed oil

Treat Small fat-free cookie

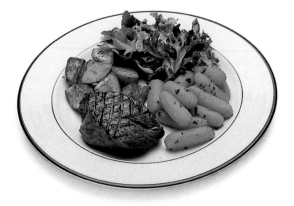

Day 6

Breakfast 1 cup low-fat yogurt mixed with ½ cup low-fat granola, 1 cup mixed berries, and 12 slivered almonds

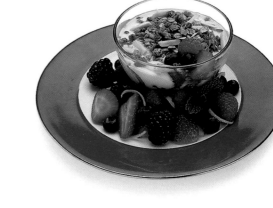

Snack 2 cups baby carrots

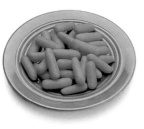

Lunch Hot dog with 1 tablespoon mustard and ketchup on bun; mixed green salad with 1 tablespoon olive oil

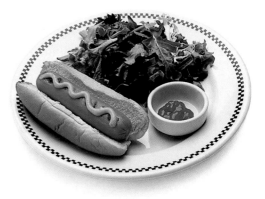

Snack 20 peanuts

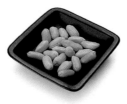

Dinner Sandwich (3 ounces grilled hamburger patty, sliced tomato and onion, 1 tablespoon ketchup, 1 tablespoon reduced-calorie mayo, served wrapped in iceberg lettuce); 10 to 15 french fries; 1 cup vegetable soup

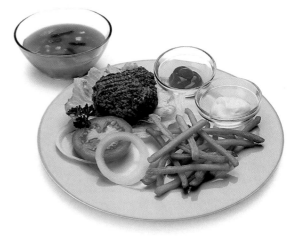

Treat 1 cup frozen seedless grapes

Day 7

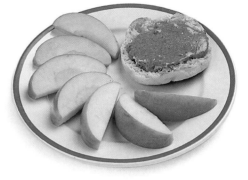

Breakfast ½ English muffin spread with 1 tablespoon almond butter; 1 sliced apple

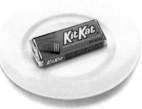

Snack 1 2-piece Kit Kat bar

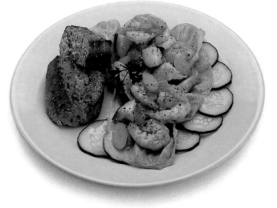

Lunch Grilled shrimp salad (3 ounces grilled shrimp, lettuce, diced tomatoes, sliced carrots, sliced cucumber, 1 tablespoon flaxseed oil); whole wheat roll

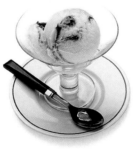

Snack ½ cup low-fat frozen yogurt

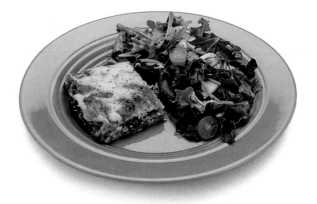

Dinner 1 square spinach lasagna; mixed green salad with 1 tablespoon flaxseed oil and chopped fresh garlic

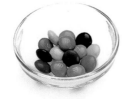

Treat ¼ small bag M&M's

cruise down plate optional food lists

As I told you in chapter 6, the Cruise Down Plate provides the simplest weight-loss method around. There's no time-consuming calorie counting. As long as you fill the top half of your plate with veggies and the bottom half with equal portions of protein and carbohydrate foods along with 1 tablespoon of fat, you will lose weight.

some suggested guidelines

I've provided the following food lists as an optional resource for those of you who want a little more security during your first week or two with the Cruise Down Plate. If you ever feel confused about how much food to place on your Cruise Down Plate, consult my simple food lists below.

Use these lists to measure out your food portions for 1 week. After that, you should be able to automatically eyeball your food portions without the need of measuring cups and spoons. Think of your first week as your week of training. Soon, you'll be ready to take off your training wheels and ride effortlessly on the road to weight loss!

protein

Consult the protein lists for specific foods, but in general, one Cruise Down Plate protein serving equals:

- 3 ounces fish, poultry, meat, or cheese (the size of a deck of cards)
- 1 cup beans
- 1 cup dairy

beans (1 cup cooked)

- Black
- Chickpeas
- Garbanzo
- Kidney
- Lentil
- Lima
- Pinto
- Refried, fat-free
- White

eggs

- 2 whole eggs
- 6 egg whites
- 1 cup egg substitute

chicken or turkey (3 ounces)

- white meat without skin
- dark meat without skin
- processed sandwich meat

seafood

fish, fresh or frozen, then grilled (3 ounces)*

- Flounder
- Halibut
- Mahimahi
- Salmon
- Sea bass
- Sole
- Swordfish
- Trout
- Tuna

*Note: If fish is fried, eat only 2 ounces.

fish, canned, packed in water

- Salmon (3 ounces)
- Sardines (4 medium)
- White tuna (albacore, 3 ounces)

shellfish (3 ounces)

- Clams
- Crab
- Crawfish
- Lobster
- Oysters (12 medium)
- Scallops

red meats (3 ounces)

- Bacon, lean (3 slices)
- Bologna (2 ounces)
- Goat
- Ham, smoked
- Hot dog, low-fat (2)
- Lamb shank or shoulder
- London broil
- Round steak
- Salami (2 ounces)
- Sausage (2 ounces)
- Sirloin steak
- Tenderloin
- Veal chop or roast

dairy

cheese, fat-free

- American (3 ounces)
- Cheddar (3 ounces)
- Cottage (1 cup)
- Feta (2 ounces)
- Monterey Jack (3 ounces)
- Mozzarella (3 ounces)
- Muenster (3 ounces)
- Parmesan, grated (4 tablespoons)
- Provolone (3 ounces)
- Ricotta (1 cup)
- Swiss (3 ounces)

milk products (1 cup)

- Lactose-free milk, low-fat, fat-free
- Milk, 1% or fat-free/skim
- Yogurt, frozen, low-fat or nonfat
- Yogurt, low-fat or nonfat

soy products

- Soybeans, cooked (1 cup)
- Soy burger (1 patty)
- Soy cheese (3 ounces)
- Soy hot dog (2)
- Soymilk (1 cup)
- Tempeh (¾ cup)
- Texturized vegetable (soy) protein (3 teaspoons or 3 ounces)
- Tofu (1 cup)

carbohydrate

Consult the carbohydrate lists for specific foods, but in general, one Cruise Down Plate carbohydrate serving equals:

- ½ cup cereal, grain, pasta, or starchy vegetables
- 1 slice bread

whole-grain breads

- Bagel, medium (½)
- Bread, reduced-calorie (2 slices)
- Bread, white, whole wheat, rye, sourdough (1 slice)
- English muffin (½)
- Hamburger or hot dog roll (½)
- Nan (unleavened bread from India, ¼ of 8" × 2" piece)
- Pita, 6-inch (½)
- Pita, 6-inch reduced-calorie (1, if less than 80 calories)
- Roll, dinner (1 small)
- Tortilla, 6-inch corn (1)
- Tortilla, 7-inch flour (1)
- Waffle, fat-free (1)

whole-grain cereals and other grains (½ cup)

- Barley, cooked
- Basmati rice, cooked
- Bran cereals
- Brown rice, cooked
- Bulgur, cooked
- Cereal, cold
- Cereal, hot
- Couscous, cooked
- Granola, low-fat
- Grits
- Jasmine rice, cooked
- Millet
- Oats

inside facts

My favorite cold cereal is Uncle Sam. It provides both whole grains and flax seeds. I eat it almost every day. Check out more about it at www.jorgecruise.com/unclesam.

- Puffed cereal (1½ cups)
- Shredded Wheat
- Sugar-frosted cereal
- Wheat germ (3 tablespoons)
- Wild rice, cooked

whole-grain pasta (½ cup)

- Spelt and millet spaghetti noodles, cooked
- Whole wheat spaghetti noodles, cooked

starchy vegetables (½ cup, count as carbs)

- Corn
- French fries (10–15)
- Potato, baked (1 small)
- Potato, mashed
- Potato, red
- Potatoes, instant
- Winter squash, acorn or butternut
- Yam/sweet potato
- Yucca root, boiled

crackers

- Animal crackers (8)
- Graham crackers (1 2½" square)
- Melba toast (4 slices)
- Oyster crackers (24)
- Potato chips, fat-free (15–20)
- Pretzels (1 ounce)
- Rice cakes (2)
- Saltine crackers (6)
- Tortilla chips, fat-free (15–20)
- Whole wheat crackers (2–5)

vegetables

Consult the vegetables list for specific foods, but in general, one Cruise Down Plate vegetable serving equals one-half of all plates.

- Artichokes
- Asparagus
- Beet greens
- Beets
- Bell peppers
- Broccoli
- Brussels sprouts
- Carrots
- Cauliflower
- Celery
- Chayote (squash)
- Collard greens
- Eggplant

- Green beans
- Kale
- Leeks
- Mung bean sprouts
- Mushrooms
- Onions
- Parsnips
- Pea pods
- Pickles (low-sodium)
- Rutabagas
- Sauerkraut
- Seaweed, raw
- Snow peas
- String beans

my favorite veggies

I love the following 12 vegetables. They are all low in calories, high in water, and delicious.

Alfalfa sprouts

Cabbage

Celery

Cucumbers

Garlic

Green onions

Jalapeños and other hot peppers

Lettuce, all types

Radishes

Spinach

Watercress

Zucchini

- Tomatillos, raw
- Tomatoes
- Tomato paste
- Tomato puree
- Tomato sauce
- Turnips
- Vegetable soups, fat-free, low-sodium

fruit

Consult the fruit lists for specific foods, but in general, one Cruise Down Plate fruit serving equals:

- One piece at breakfast or as a snack
- Lemons and limes are unlimited (they do not count)

limited fruits

- Apple, green or red (1 medium)
- Applesauce, unsweetened (½ cup)
- Apricots (4)
- Banana, 5-inch (1)
- Blackberries (¾ cup)
- Blueberries (¾ cup)
- Cantaloupe (⅓ melon or 1 cup cubed)
- Cherries (12 large)
- Dates (3)
- Figs, dried (1)
- Figs, fresh (2 medium)
- Fruit cocktail (½ cup)

- Grapefruit (½)
- Grapes, green or red (12)
- Honeydew (⅓ melon or 1 cup cubed)
- Kiwi (1 large)
- Mango (1 small)
- Orange (1 medium)
- Papaya (1 cup cubed)
- Peach (1 medium)
- Pear, green (1 small)
- Pineapple, canned, packed in juice (⅓ cup)
- Plums (2 medium)
- Prunes (2)
- Raisins (2 tablespoons)
- Raspberries (1 cup)
- Strawberries (1 cup)
- Watermelon (1 cup cubed)

fruit juice (½ cup)

- Apple juice/cider
- Cranberry juice
- Grapefruit juice
- Orange juice
- Pineapple juice

fat

Consult the fat lists for specific foods, but in general, one Cruise Down Plate fat serving equals:

- 1 tablespoon oil
- 12 nuts

preferred fats

- Almond butter (1 tablespoon)
- Almonds (12)
- Avocado (¼ or 2 ounces)
- Cashews (12)
- Extra-virgin olive oil (1 tablespoon)
- Flaxseed oil (1 tablespoon)
- Oil-based salad dressing (2 tablespoons)
- Olives (10)
- Peanut butter (1 tablespoon)
- Peanuts (20)
- Pecans (8 halves)
- Pumpkin seeds (2 tablespoons)
- Sesame seeds (2 tablespoons)
- Soy mayonnaise (2 tablespoons)
- Sunflower seeds (2 tablespoons)

fats to minimize

- Butter, reduced-calorie (1 tablespoon)
- Butter, stick (2 teaspoons)

critical secrets

In order to get 1 tablespoon of flaxseed oil from a supplement, you must use eight capsules. If you squeeze the oil out of the eight capsules, it will equal 1 tablespoon.

- Butter, whipped (2 teaspoons)
- Coconut, shredded
  (4 tablespoons)
- Corn oil (2 teaspoons)
- Cream cheese, reduced-calorie
  (2 tablespoons)
- Half-and-half (2 tablespoons)
- Mayonnaise (1 teaspoon)
- Mayonnaise, reduced-calorie
  (1 tablespoon)
- Safflower oil (2 teaspoons)
- Shortening (1 teaspoon)
- Sour cream, reduced-calorie
  (2 tablespoons)
- Soybean oil (2 teaspoons)

snacks

In general, your snacks should be about 100 calories. Consult the snacks list for specific portion sizes.

- Almonds (12)
- Angle food cake (2-ounce slice)
- Baby carrots (2 cups)
- Baker's cookie
  (www.bbcookies.com) (1)
- Brownie (1)
- Butterscotch (4 pieces)
- Candy corn (20 pieces)
- Cashews (12)
- Celery (3 sticks with 1 teaspoon
  of peanut butter on each)
- Chocolate-covered almonds (7)
- Fruit, 1 piece (see fruit lists for
  portion size)

- Fudge (1 ounce)
- Gelatin (½ cup)
- GeniSoy Soy Crisps (25)
- Granola bar, low-fat (1)
- Gumdrops (1 ounce)
- Heath bar (1 snack size)
- Hershey's milk chocolate bar
  (1 small)
- Hershey's milk chocolate bar
  with almonds (1 small)
- Hershey's Sweet Escapes
  (1 bar, any kind)
- Kit Kat (1 2-piece bar)
- Kudos with M&M's granola
  bar (1)
- Melba toast (4 slices)
- No Pudge! Fat Free Fudge
  Brownie (www.nopudge.com)
  (1 2" square)
- Oyster crackers (24)
- Peanut brittle (1 ounce)
- Peanuts (20)
- Pecans (8 halves)
- Popcorn, air popped (1 cup)
- Potato chips, fat-free (15–20)
- Pound cake (1-ounce slice)
- Pretzels (¾ ounce)
- Pudding cup, fat-free (1)
- Pumpkin seeds (2 tablespoons)
- Raisins (30)
- Rice cakes (2)
- Saltine crackers (6)
- Sesame seeds (2 tablespoons)

- Sherbet (½ cup)
- Skinny Cow fat-free fudge bar
  (1)
- Skinny Cow low-fat ice cream
  sandwich (½)
- String cheese (1)
- Sunflower seeds
  (2 tablespoons)
- Tofutti (¼ cup)
- Tortilla chips, fat-free (15–20)
- Uncle Sam Cereal
  (½ cup dry)
- Whole wheat crackers (2–5)
- Whoppers malted milk balls
  (9)
- Yogurt, frozen, low-fat or
  nonfat (½ cup)
- Yogurt, low-fat or nonfat
  (8 ounces)

treats

Eat a delicious treat every day. In general, they should be up to 50 calories. Consult the treats list for specific portion sizes.

- Cheese slice, reduced-calorie
  (1)
- Chocolate chips (½ tablespoon)
- Chocolate-coated mints (4)
- Cookie, fat-free (1 small)
- Cranberry sauce (¼ cup)
- Frozen seedless grapes
  (1 cup)
- Gelatin dessert, sugar-free (1)

- Gingersnaps (3)
- Graham crackers (1 2½" square)
- Gumdrops (8 small)
- Hard candy (1)
- Hershey's Hugs or Kisses (2)
- Hershey's Miniatures (1, any kind)
- Jelly beans (7)
- Licorice twist (1)
- Oreo cookie (1)
- Marshmallow (1 large)
- M&M's (¼ of small bag)
- M&M's Minis (¼ of tube)
- Miss Meringue cookie (www.missmeringue.com) (1)
- Nonfat ice cream (½ cup) drizzled with Hershey's chocolate syrup
- Popcorn, air popped (1 cup)
- Reese's Peanut Butter Cup (1)

alcohol

I recommend you cut back or omit alcohol due to its high caloric content. If you decide to splurge for a special occasion, though, substitute alcohol for one of your daily snacks and hold yourself to one drink, such as:

- a 12-ounce light beer
- a 5-ounce glass of wine
- 1½ ounces of liquor

- SnackWell's sandwich cookie (1)
- York peppermint pattie (1 small)

freebies

The following items equal one Cruise Down Plate freebie. Consume them as often as you like.

drinks

- Canarino Italian hot lemon drink (www.canarino.com)
- Carbonated or mineral water (Add lime or lemon for great taste!)
- Decaffeinated coffee, plain
- Green or herbal tea
- Soft drinks, calorie-free

seasonings

- Garlic
- Herbs, fresh or dried
- Kernel Season's Gourmet Popcorn Seasoning (www.kernel seasons.com—also excellent on pasta, vegetables, chicken, potatoes, eggs, and pitas!)
- Mrs. Dash
- Nonstick cooking spray
- Pimiento
- Salsas, Tabasco, or hot pepper sauce
- Spices

your questions

Mustard is a freebie, but what about ketchup?

Try to limit your use of ketchup to 1 tablespoon due to its higher sugar content.

condiments

- Horseradish
- Lemon juice
- Lime juice
- Mustard
- Soy sauce, light
- Vinegar
- Walden Farms salad dressings (www.waldenfarms.com)

sugar substitutes

- Splenda (www.splenda.com)
- Sugar-free chewing gum
- SweetLeaf stevia products (www.steviaplus.com)

Photocopy this page and carry it with you. Date it and start with Step 1. Then move to Step 2 and log your Cruise Moves. During the day, write down what you eat in Step 3 and check off your glasses of water. Don't forget your snacks and treat.

THE CRUISE
WEIGHT-LOSS PLANNER

Date _____

Step 1: Before the 8 Minutes—The People Solution

☐ Check here once you have completed today's activity.

Step 2: The 8 Minutes—Cruise Moves

	Move Name	Set 1 (✔)	Set 2 (✔)	Set 3 (✔)	Set 4 (✔)
A					
B					

Step 3: After the 8 Minutes—Cruise Down Plate

Breakfast

Veggies/Fruit _____

Carbs _____

Protein _____

Fat _____

Snack

Lunch

Veggies _____

Carbs _____

Protein _____

Fat _____

Snack

Dinner

Veggies _____

Carbs _____

Protein _____

Fat _____

Treat

Water (✔): ○ ○ ○ ○ ○ ○ ○ ○

become a weight-loss star

Here's a motivational incentive to keep you going. After you reach your goal weight, send me your weight-loss success story. Doing so will put you in the running to qualify to meet me in person in an all-expenses-paid trip to beautiful San Diego!

Plus, if you are selected, I might feature you during my television appearances, in my magazine columns, on my Web site, or in upcoming books. You'll become a weight-loss star across the nation.

Here's how it works. Each year, I host a red rose ceremony in San Diego for my most inspirational and successful clients. With help from my staff, I pick 20 people for the yearly trip. You'll receive a free makeover, new wardrobe, and VIP maintenance plan designed exclusively for you (a $10,000 value). At the ceremony, I will recognize you in front of an auditorium filled with more than 200 people. We will capture the event on camera so I can share your amazing success story with all of America. So, are you ready to become an inspirational role model to millions?

how to apply

Visit www.jorgecruise.com/red rose and download the Red Rose Success Story form. Fill it out and mail it, along with your "before" and "after" photos, to the address listed on the form.

Good luck and best wishes!

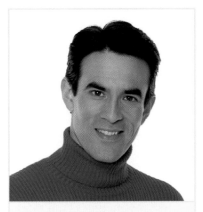

"Putting your body first gives you the health and energy you need to live your life to its fullest."

the synergy page

ready for more?

Check out these synergistic ways to take the 8-minute plan to the next level.

jorgecruise.com: the #1 weight-loss club for busy people

To be truly successful at weight loss, you must also connect with others. Trying to lose weight alone is a formula for failure. The need to talk with others who are also losing weight is very important. This need to connect is sometimes even more important than the need to lose weight. Bottom line: You must get encouragement and support. Weight-loss desires company, and the *all-new* JorgeCruise.com Web site will provide you the undying support you require.

At JorgeCruise.com, you'll discover many exciting things:

- Daily messages from me
- Weekly online meetings
- Live chat auditoriums with me
- Expert advice from my weight-loss mentors
- Tools to chart your weight loss
- And much more . . .

Joining my *all-new* online weight-loss club is like joining a family!

the video system

Personally experience my dynamic coaching style in your own home!

With this high-energy video, you will feel that you are shoulder-to-shoulder with me, your weight-loss coach. I will walk you through, step-by-step, 1 week's worth of my superquick 8-minute moves. It could not be easier. For more information, go to www.jorgecruise.com/videosystem, but look at what my video offers:

- The ideal next step to this book
- No special equipment required
- Motivating and energetic music to make it more fun

cruise down® flax oil

Curb your appetite and make weight loss even easier.

My Cruise Down Flax Oil is an all-natural omega-3 liquid complex that helps control your hunger and tastes great on food. Use as a salad dressing, mixed with yogurt, shakes, on toast in the morning, and much more!

Just a tablespoon with each meal, and you will shrink your appetite away. It's also available in capsule form. For more information, go to www.jorgecruise.com/flaxoil, but check out the best part about my Cruise Down Flax Oil:

- Satisfies your hunger so you won't overeat
- Absolutely no stimulants
- Includes the natural fat-burning enzyme lipase

prevention magazine column

Get inspired every month by reading real-life success stories in my new column, "The Weight Loss Coach," in *Prevention* magazine.

Dramatic "before" and "after" photos of people just like you will keep you motivated to stick with the program. You'll learn their secrets for success and tips for overcoming everyday obstacles. Whether it's emotional eating, a busy lifestyle, or a lack of confidence that's sidetracking your efforts, "The Weight Loss Coach" will get you back on the right track. So join me and discover how you can slim down, shape up, and get healthy.

About the Author

Jorge Cruise: America's #1 Online Weight-Loss Specialist

Jorge (pronounced HOR-hay) Cruise is the *New York Times* best-selling author of *8 Minutes in the Morning*® and is recognized as the number-one *online* weight-loss specialist, due to his unprecedented success in helping more than 3 million people lose weight at his Web site, JorgeCruise.com.

Jorge has been featured in the *New York Times*, *USA Today*, *People*, *Woman's World*, *First for Women*, *Self*, *Shape*, *Cosmopolitan*, and *Fit* and has appeared on *Oprah*, CNN, *Good Morning America*, *Dateline*, *Extra*, and Lifetime Television.

No other weight-loss specialist has had so many people directly reveal what really works at consistently losing 2 pounds each week in just 8 minutes. This makes Jorge one of the most up-to-date and in-demand weight-loss specialists both online and off.

Jorge is also a nominee for Fitness Instructor of the Year by IDEA, the national association of fitness professionals, and was named by Arnold Schwarzenegger as a special advisor to the California Governor's Council on Physical Fitness and Sports.

In addition, 11 million people read his monthly column, "The Weight Loss Coach," in *Prevention* magazine. Jorge is also a member of the Association of Health Care Journalists, a nonprofit organization dedicated to advancing public understanding of health care issues. He is fluent in both English and Spanish.

Utilizing the knowledge and credentials that he has gained from the University of California, San Diego, Dartmouth College, the Cooper Institute for Aerobics Research, the American College of Sports Medicine, and the American Council on Exercise, Jorge is dedicated to helping time-deprived women, men, kids, and seniors lose weight and achieve their dreams.

He lives in San Diego with his wife, Heather. He can be contacted via www.JorgeCruise.com.

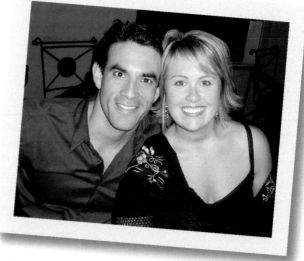

Me and my girl, Heather